A Simple Guide to Trauma

R. L. Huckstep CMG FTS

MA MD(Cantab) FRCS(Edin) FRCS(Eng) FRACS

Professor and Head, Department of Traumatic and Orthopaedic
Surgery and Chairman, School of Surgery, University of New
South Wales, Sydney, Australia; Chairman of Orthopaedic
Surgery and Director of Accident Services, Prince of Wales and
Prince Henry Hospitals, Sydney, Australia; Chairman or
Member, various Accident and Disaster Committees in Australia
and Senior Medical Disaster Commander, Sydney, Australia;
Corresponding Editor, Injury and Archives of Orthopaedic and
Traumatic Surgery; *Lately* Vice-President, Australian
Orthopaedic Association; Professor of Orthopaedic Surgery,
Makerere University, Kampala, Uganda; Hunterian Professor,
Royal College of Surgeons of England; Corresponding Editor,
Journal of Bone and Joint Surgery

ILLUSTRATIONS BY

W. Serumaga

DFA CertMI(London) MMAA AIMBI

Head of the Medical Illustration Department, Makerere
University, Kampala, Uganda, East Africa

Franca Rubiu

Lately Medical Artist, University of New South Wales, Sydney,
Australia

J. D. Greenstein

BSc MB BS(NSW)

Medical Practitioner, Sydney, Australia

FOURTH EDITION

CHURCHILL LIVINGSTONE

EDINBURGH LONDON MELBOURNE AND NEW YORK 1986

CHURCHILL LIVINGSTONE
Medical Division of Longman Group UK Limited

Distributed in the United States of America by Churchill
Livingstone Inc., 1560 Broadway, New York, N.Y. 10036, and
by associated companies, branches and representatives
throughout the world.

First Edition 1970
    Reprinted 1972
    Reprinted 1974
Italian Edition 1975
Second Edition 1978
    Reprinted 1979
Third Edition 1982
    Reprinted 1983
Japanese Edition 1983
Fourth Edition 1986

ISBN 0 443 03350 1

British Library Cataloguing in Publication Data
Huckstep, R. L.
    A simple guide to trauma—4th ed.
    1. Wounds and injuries—Treatment
    2. Medical emergencies
    I. Title II. Serumaga, W. III. Rubiu,
    Franca IV. Greenstein, J. D.
    617'.1026 RD93

Library of Congress Cataloging in Publication Data
Huckstep, R. L. (Ronald Lawrie)
    A simple guide to trauma

    Bibliography: p.
    Includes index.
    1. Wounds and injuries. 2. First aid in illness and
injuries. I. Title. [DNLM: 1. Emergencies—handbooks.
2. Wounds and Injuries—handbooks. WO 39 H882s]
    RD93.H9 1986 617'.1 86-9588

Produced by Longman Singapore Publishers (Pte) Ltd.
Printed in Singapore.

Preface

Since the publication of the first three editions there has been a continuing heavy demand for this book, from medical and paramedical personnel, particularly those working in Casualty and Accident Departments and in various rescue organisations. This situation has necessitated several reprints, together with Italian and Japanese editions.

It is felt that this book could prove of value, not only to medical students and doctors, but also to nurses, ambulance officers, physiotherapists and those trained in first aid. Those requiring a first aid manual and more details about the management of injuries should also find it useful.

In this fourth edition many advances in the treatment of injuries have been incorporated in the text, and nearly every page has been brought up to date and the printing has been considerably improved. The text and illustrations are based on six previous editions of *A Simple Guide to Injuries*, reprinted many times during the past twenty five years, and on the first three editions of *A Simple Guide to Trauma*. This book has thus combined both books in a simple monograph still small enough to be carried in a white coat pocket or the glove box of a car and to this end it has been slightly reduced in overall size, in spite of a slightly increased content.

Although the most modern methods of management of injuries are advocated in these pages the accent is always, as in the first three editions, on basic, safe, standard, proven methods of treatment with, I hope, a balance between the new and the well tried. The emphasis, however, has been on simplicity, and the latest methods of splinting and internal fixation, in order that the patient should be mobile and out of bed as soon as possible. Skelecasts and simple aluminium splints, which have proved effective in several thousand cases by the author, are particularly important in this regard. The use of these, plus crepe bandages and early movements, has meant that many patients can be mobilised early and can often return to work much earlier than with heavy hot plasters. Similarly, the modern methods of internal fixation of fractures will often mean much earlier mobility and discharge from hospital. Only the most important and relevant details of patient management are included because of the need to keep the book small. On the other hand, a few operative details of emergency care, such as amputations and vascular compression in supracondylar fractures, are included for the doctor working in an isolated hospital or in a developing country where there may be minimal assistance.

I should like to thank Mrs Franca Rubiu and Dr James Greenstein for updating many of the illustrations, as well as drawing new ones. These complement Mr Serumaga's original illustrations.

My thanks are also due to Mr Frank Strmecki for his help with the lettering and to members of the Medical Illustration Department of the University of New South Wales, particularly Mr K. Deason and Mr Michael Oakey who have been most helpful in photographing the pages.

I am also grateful to the late Dr Hugh Smith whose help and encouragement enabled the development of many new inventions in the Hugh Smith Orthopaedic Research Department of the University of New South Wales.

I am indebted to Professors R. F. Jones and T. Torda, Drs M. A. R. Baldwin, E. H. Bates, G. K. Bruce, B. G. Courtenay, M. J. Donnellan, J. E. Frawley, A. Gonski, L. Gray, R. G. Macbeth, V. J. Mansberg, R. McGuinness, A. McJannet, W. Walsh and I. Woodforth for their help and advice in various specialised sections of the book, as well as to the members of the Department of Traumatic and Orthopaedic Surgery and the surgeons of the University of New South Wales for their constructive suggestions.

I should also particularly like to thank Miss Julie Bown and Mrs Mitzi Bourne for typing the manuscript. I should like to thank Miss Jackie Curtis, Mr M. A. Davies, Mrs Dawn Dennis, Mrs Renee Hannan, Miss Danielle Hannan, Michael and Nigel Huckstep, Miss Susan Huckstep, Mrs Ulla Hudson, Mrs Maree Jordan, Mr J. H. Lee, Mrs Judith Lynch, Miss Judith Mountford, Mr G. Rice-McDonald,

Mr G. Swavley as well as Drs A. Beveridge, G. Cameron, G. Fettke, J. Fuller, R. Piper, S. Riordan and M. Tiutiunnik for their help.

I am also grateful to the staff of Churchill Livingstone for their unfailing courtesy and assistance in the production of this edition, and to the manager of Frontier Technology Pty Ltd, Mr J. Murray, and his staff, especially Mrs Sue Corvisy, for their help in printing the text.

Finally, as in all previous editions, I should like to thank my wife for checking and editing the manuscript.

Sydney, 1986   R. L. Huckstep

Contents

Upper limb

Spine

Pelvis

Lower limb

Post-operative care

ABBREVIATIONS
P = Physiotherapy   S = Surgery

EMERGENCY MANAGEMENT

FIRST AID AND EMERGENCY MANAGEMENT SUMMARY

PRIORITIES

1. **Clear Airway.** Position patient - Mouth to mouth resuscitation External cardiac massage.
2. **Stop Bleeding.** Elevate and splint limb.
3. **Resuscitate patient.** Treat other injuries.

RESPIRATORY OBSTRUCTION AND SHOCK

1. Patient on **side** if semi-conscious or unconscious. Maintain airway. Give oxygen.
2. Elevate foot of bed, (not in head and chest injuries) or patient's feet. Do NOT over heat patient.
3. Morphia **intravenously** for pain — if **no** contra-indications such as head injury or respiratory arrest. Put up I.V. drip.

HAEMORRHAGE

1. Elevate feet, but do not tilt head down. Elevate bleeding limb.
2. **Local** pressure by wool and bandage direct on bleeding point. Avoid tourniquet.
3. Group specific blood if available. S.P.P.S. or plasma expander if NO blood.

VISCERAL INJURIES

1. **Damage** to lung leading to:
   (a) Pneumothorax ⎫ Urgent aspiration
   (b) Haemothorax ⎬ or closed
   (c) Haemopneumothorax ⎭ drainage
2. **Damage to Heart and Pericardium**
   Cardiac tamponade — Urgent aspiration. Treat arrhythmias, if present.
3. **Damage to Abdominal Viscera -**
   Many are under ribs — See abdominal injuries.

FIRST AID
PRINCIPLES
KEEP PATIENT ALIVE
SPEED <u>NOT</u> STERILITY

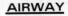 **AIRWAY**

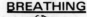 **BREATHING**

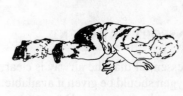

Clear   Oropharynx

Patient On Side

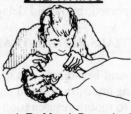

Mouth To Mouth Resuscitation

If Necessary

<u>NEVER LEAVE</u>
<u>AN UNCONSCIOUS PATIENT UNATTENDED ON BACK</u>

CIRC<u>ULATION</u>

Arms Straight

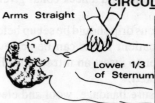

Lower 1/3
of Sternum

CARDIAC MASSAGE

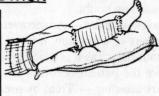

STOP BLEEDING ELEVATE

LIMB

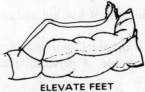

ELEVATE FEET

TREAT SHOCK

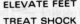
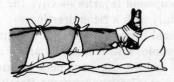

SPLINT FRACTURES
Check Pulse and Capillary Return

EMERGENCY TRANSPORT IN SEVERE INJURIES

Severely injured patients must be transported to the nearest **suitable** hospital able to treat the patient, rather than to the nearest hospital. Resuscitate and give first aid before the patient is transported, but avoid delay.

ESSENTIALS BEFORE TRANSPORT OF PATIENT

Airway and breathing — It is essential that the airway is clear, breathing unobstructed and oxygen should be given if available. Mouth to mouth resuscitation may be necessary. Do not transport unless breathing is ensured.

Unconscious Patients — Unconscious patients should be nursed on the side in the "coma" position. Care must be taken with a possible fracture of the cervical spine, and a neck collar given if there is any doubt.

Intravenous Fluid — An intravenous drip should be set up before transport of a severely injured patient if this can be achieved without delay, as it is much easier to insert an intravenous line before the patient becomes shocked.

Severe bleeding — Treat by pressure bandage, wool and elevation before transport, plus an IV plasma expander.

Fractures — Tie the two legs together or splint fractures by the other methods illustrated.

Compound Injuries — Give the simplest of first aid and cover lightly with a clean dressing.

Spinal Injuries — Keep a patient with spinal injuries as flat as possible. Use a spinal board if available. A cervical collar is needed for suspected neck injuries.

Communications with the Receiving Hospital — The hospital should be informed about the type of injury.

EMERGENCY TRANSPORT

HOSPITAL

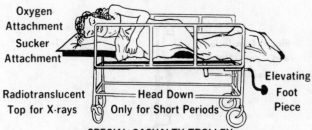

Oxygen Attachment
Sucker Attachment

Elevating Foot Piece

Radiotranslucent Top for X-rays — Head Down — Only for Short Periods

SPECIAL CASUALTY TROLLEY
CASUALTY TROLLEY MUST HAVE SIDE RAILS

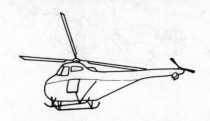

HELICOPTER WHEN POSSIBLE

Well Padded Back Slab | Modified Thomas Splint

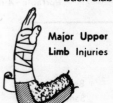
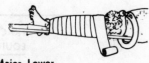

Major Upper Limb Injuries

Major Lower Limb Injuries
Bandage or Plaster Over Wool

SPLINTING FOR TRAVEL

EMERGENCY RECEPTION

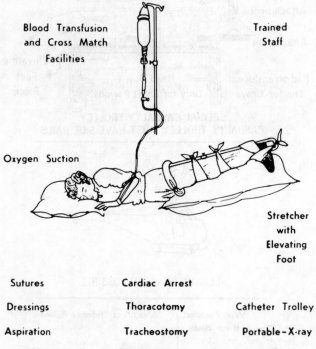

Blood Transfusion
and Cross Match
Facilities

Trained
Staff

Oxygen Suction

Stretcher
with
Elevating
Foot

Sutures	Cardiac Arrest	
Dressings	Thoracotomy	Catheter Trolley
Aspiration	Tracheostomy	Portable - X-ray

FRACTURE
EQUIPMENT

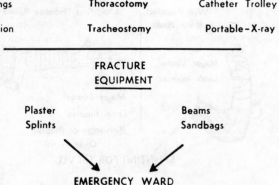

Plaster
Splints

Beams
Sandbags

EMERGENCY WARD

EMERGENCY THEATRE

Anaesthetic Equipment and Suction

Cardiac Arrest
Thoracotomy
Tracheostomy

Catheterisation
Laparotomy
Craniotomy

Cardiac Arrest Trolley

C.V.P. MONITOR AND I.V. DRIP

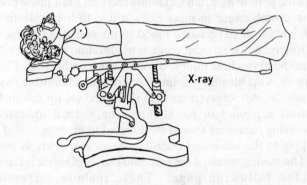

X-ray

EMERGENCY DRUGS

Adrenaline
Metaraminol
Hydrocortisone
Atropine
Calcium Gluconate
Potassium Chloride
Lignocaine
Sodium Bicarbonate

Antibiotics
Analgesics
Sedatives
T.I.G.
Toxoid

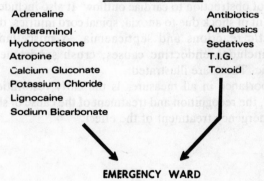

EMERGENCY WARD

SHOCK

The management of shock in the injured patient can be divided into immediate life saving measures, diagnosis, management of the cause and long-term treatment.

The typical picture of the shocked patient is illustrated, and the patient may be conscious or unconscious. The pulse is usually rapid and weak (compared with slow and bounding in fainting) and the patient pale, cold, clammy and with a **low blood pressure.** The overall cause in most cases is due to hypovolaemia with diminution of oxygenated blood to the essential organs.

Emergency treatment consists of elevation of the feet if there is no head or chest injury, or other contraindication. Clear the airway, stop bleeding, splint fracture and administer oxygen if available. An intravenous drip should be set up routinely and plasma expander or blood should be given if indicated. All lifesaving measures should be directed to an oxygenated blood supply to the brain and essential organs as quickly as possible.

The management of the common causes of shock is illustrated in the following pages. These include correction of hypovolaemia due to bleeding, the management of cardiogenic shock and of obstruction to cardiac outflow. It also includes the management of shock due to anoxia, spinal cord injuries, drugs, anaphylactic reactions and septicaemia. A miscellaneous category includes endocrine causes, crush syndrome and psychogenic. These are illustrated.

The importance in all measures is the early restoration of circulation, the recognition and treatment of the cause of shock, and the emergency treatment of the effect.

SHOCK
FIRST AID
INITIAL ASSESSMENT

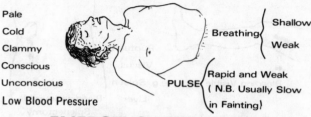

Pale
Cold
Clammy
Conscious
Unconscious
Low Blood Pressure

Breathing { Shallow / Weak

PULSE { Rapid and Weak (N.B. Usually Slow in Fainting)

EMERGENCY TREATMENT

CLEAR AIRWAY   CONTROL BLEEDING   Elevate Feet
   Loosen Collar   DIRECT PRESSURE   Splint Fractures
   One Pillow   Cover Burns

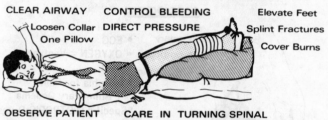

OBSERVE PATIENT   CARE IN TURNING SPINAL
                       AND NECK INJURIES

OXYGEN

Hydrostatic Inflatable
Trousers for Shock

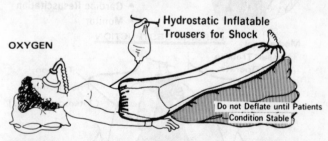

Do not Deflate until Patients
Condition Stable

RESTORE
CIRCULATION —Intravenous Drip— { - Hartmanns - Haemaccel
                                   - SPPS - Dextran Plasma
                                   - Blood   Expanders
DETAILED ASSESSMENT AND TREAT CAUSE
Analgesics and Drugs ONLY if necessary
and then Intravenously

SHOCK
CAUSES
HYPOVOLAEMIA

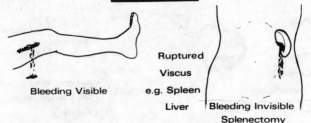

Bleeding Visible

Ruptured
Viscus
e.g. Spleen
Liver

Bleeding Invisible
Splenectomy

STOP BLEEDING - REPLACE BLOOD VOLUME

CARDIOGENIC

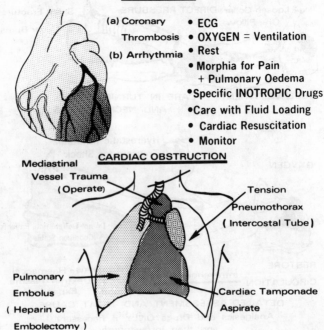

(a) Coronary
Thrombosis

(b) Arrhythmia

- ECG
- OXYGEN = Ventilation
- Rest
- Morphia for Pain
  + Pulmonary Oedema
- Specific INOTROPIC Drugs
- Care with Fluid Loading
- Cardiac Resuscitation
- Monitor

CARDIAC OBSTRUCTION

Mediastinal
Vessel Trauma
(Operate)

Tension
Pneumothorax
(Intercostal Tube)

Pulmonary
Embolus
(Heparin or
Embolectomy)

Cardiac Tamponade
Aspirate

SHOCK

DRUGS AND ANAPHYLACTIC

I.V. Fluids

Adrenaline

Corticosteroids

Respiratory and Cardiac Stimulants

Renal Dialysis   Antidotes

Treat Cause

SPINAL CORD INJURY

Plasma Volume Expanders
and Vasoconstrictors
Inotropic Drugs
in small doses

SEPTICAEMIA

Bacterial ⌐ Intravenous
            Fluids
         ├ Antibiotics and
Adrenal   Corticosteroids
Failure ⌐

ANOXIA

Cerebral and ⌐ Airway
Cardiac   Oxygen
Ischaemia ⌐ Blood

ENDOCRINE

Addisonian ⌐ Fluids
Crisis   Steroids

Treat Cause

MISCELLANEOUS

Crush Syndrome

Post Traumatic Syndrome

? Amputate if More Than
6 hours Severe Crush
+
I.V. Fluids
+
Oxygen

PSYCHOGENIC CAUSES MAY ALSO BE PRESENT — TREAT

INTRAVENOUS INFUSION

It is essential that an intravenous infusion be set up quickly in a severely injured or shocked patient. This should be done at the accident site **before** the patient has become shocked further and veins become difficult to find. If there is difficulty in finding the vein, or if the resuscitator is unskilled, the patient should be transported to hospital **without** delay.

A fairly wide gauge needle (size 14 or 16) should be used wherever possible in the veins in the forearm, as illustrated. The butterfly needle is only used for giving drugs or if a larger needle cannot be inserted.

A plastic blood or IV fluid container should be used at the site of accident, as it can be compressed and used as a pressure pump to speed up tranfusion. This is of particular value in a mining or crush injury in confined spaces when fluid has to be pumped into the vein with little hydrostatic height available.

A central venous line (in the subclavian or jugular vein) should be inserted in hospital in a **severely** shocked patient for assessing the central venous pressure and giving fluids.

Normal saline or Ringer solution should be used to set up the drip but this should be followed in shocked patients by S.P.P.S. or another plasma expander, until blood is available.

In shock the patient's feet should be elevated as soon as possible or hydrostatic inflatable trousers applied, but do not tilt head down. These compress the lower limbs and abdomen with a safety valve to prevent over-inflation. These can return about 1 to 1.5 litres of blood to the circulation. It is essential that the compartments be released **gradually** to each leg and the abdomen and pelvis, and **only** after shock has been combatted.

INTRAVENOUS INFUSION

APPARATUS

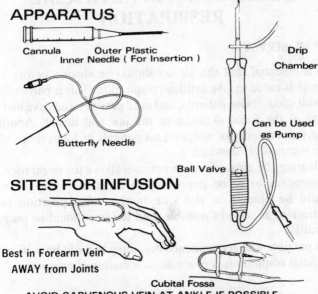

Cannula   Outer Plastic
   Inner Needle (For Insertion)

Drip

Chamber

Can be Used
as Pump

Butterfly Needle

Ball Valve

SITES FOR INFUSION

Best in Forearm Vein
AWAY from Joints

Cubital Fossa

AVOID SAPHENOUS VEIN AT ANKLE IF POSSIBLE
USE HYDROSTATIC INFLATABLE TROUSERS
IN SEVERE SHOCK

CENTRAL VENOUS PRESSURE

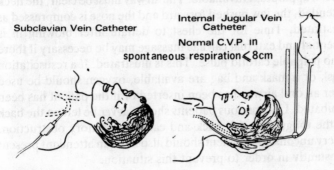

Subclavian Vein Catheter

Internal Jugular Vein
Catheter

Normal C.V.P. in
spontaneous respiration < 8cm

INSTRUCTION IN ARTIFICIAL RESPIRATION

CLEAR AIRWAY

It is essential that the airway should be cleared before any attempt is made to give artificial respiration. This is particularly so in all unconscious patients, and in all patients who have had an injury of the facial skeleton or the jaw and throat. Another important category of unconscious patients includes those who have vomited or drowned.

Clearing the airway in such patients allows for respiration to recommence or to be improved. In these cases the patients should be placed on the side in the coma position (see illustration) as soon as possible, and the jaw should be pushed forward.

In patients who recommence breathing this will be sufficient. Artificial respiration is essential as a matter of urgency.

ARTIFICIAL RESPIRATION

Mouth to mouth resuscitation is by far the best method if no special apparatus is available. The airway must be clear, the neck extended, the jaw pushed forward and the nose is compressed as illustrated. Time for the chest to deflate after blowing in is essential and external cardiac massage may be necessary if there is no palpable carotid pulse. This is illustrated. If a resuscitation mask or a mask and bag are available, oxygen should be used after an oral airway has been inserted or if the patient has been intubated. Unconscious patients should **never** be left on the back as the tongue can fall back and cause respiratory obstruction. Every unconscious patient should also have an attendant present constantly in order to prevent this situation.

EMERGENCY RESPIRATION
MECHANISM OF OBSTRUCTION

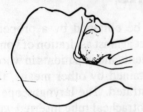 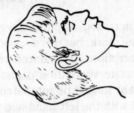

Tongue Falls Back and Obstructs Airway

INITIAL TREATMENT

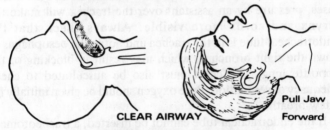

CLEAR AIRWAY

Pull Jaw Forward

FURTHER TREATMENT

Posture on Side to Prevent
Inhalation of Vomitus
and Keep Tongue Forward

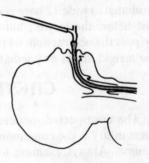

If Unable to Maintain Airway
Insert Oral Airway
or Endotracheal Tube

<u>**NEVER LEAVE**</u>
<u>**AN UNCONSCIOUS PATIENT**</u>
<u>**UNATTENDED ON HIS BACK**</u>

Airway or
Endotracheal Tube

RESPIRATORY ASSISTANCE IN HOSPITAL

Increased inspired oxygen can be obtained by a properly fitting mask, but this does not protect against aspiration of vomit or secretions. In an unconscious patient, and in patients in whom adequate ventilation cannot be obtained by other means, the patient should be intubated as illustrated. The laryngoscope is held with the left hand and the endotracheal tube inserted with the right after dentures have been removed, and the throat cleared of secretions. The tongue is lifted forward and in difficult cases, pressure by an assistant over the trachea will make the larynx and cords more visible. Always check that the endotracheal tube is in the trachea and not in the oesophagus or down the right bronchus, which may result in blocking of the opposite lung. The chest must also be auscultated to check adequacy of ventilation. Pure oxygen should be given initially for a few breaths.

If the endotracheal tube cannot be inserted, a tracheotome is preferable to a tracheostomy. As an immediate measure, in the case of patients with severe facial injuries who cannot be intubated, a wide 12 bore needle can be inserted into the trachea just below the larynx, but only as an emergency measure to by-pass the obstruction, or probably the best way to do this is to use a rigid infant or paediatric bronchoscope.

CHEST INJURIES

The unsuspected, underestimated and inadequately treated chest injury is the commonest cause of preventable death from trauma. Always examine for damage to the **lung** and **pleura, heart** and **pericardium, ribs** and **sternum, oesophagus** and **diaphragm** and **major vessels.** Compression injuries can cause major internal injury with minor damage to chest wall. Beware progressive anoxia from lung contusion.

EMERGENCY RESPIRATION
APNOEA-ARTIFICIAL VENTILATION

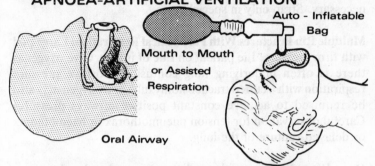

Auto - Inflatable Bag

Mouth to Mouth or Assisted Respiration

Oral Airway

ENDOTRACHEAL INTUBATION

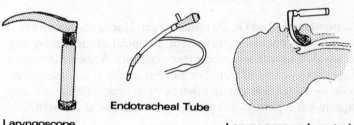

Endotracheal Tube

Laryngoscope

Laryngoscope Inserted

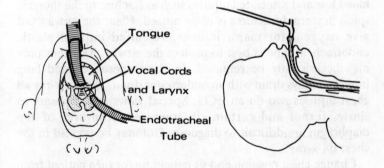

Tongue

Vocal Cords and Larynx

Endotracheal Tube

Minor Rib Fractures: Injection of local anaesthetic only if necessary. Strap **only** in special cases.

Multiple Rib Fractures With Paradoxical Respiration: Large pad with firm pressure. Lie patient on side of injury. Give oxygen as there is often underlying lung contusion. Positive pressure respiration with a cuffed tracheostomy tube and oxygen may also be required to achieve constant positive airways pressure. Careful observation for tension pneumothorax or haemothorax or delayed rupture of the lung.

Open Wounds: Close with vaseline gauze and pad and aspirate air or blood. Always use an underwater drain in hospital plus prophylactic chemotherapy.

Haemothorax And/Or Pneumothorax: Haemothorax needs a basal drain, pneumothorax needs an apical drain. Emergency removal of air with any needle (see diagram). A needle through a finger stall or end of a rubber glove is useful in an emergency. **Note** — A tension pneumothorax or cardiac tamponade may rapidly kill a patient if not diagnosed and quickly treated.

General — Always treat the patient as well as the injury. **Shock, blood loss** and associated injuries such as fracture of the thoracic spine in sternal fractures is often missed. Clear the airway and give oxygen, for major injuries. A cuffed inflated plastic endotracheal tube is best to protect the airway. Tracheostomy may occasionally be required. In chest operations and lung injuries always drain with an underwater drain. Always x-ray **all** chest injuries and do an ECG. Special views are necessary to show sternal and certain rib fractures. Ruptures of the diaphragm are difficult to diagnose. Gut may be present in the chest on x-ray.

Change chest position and sit patient up, or turn patient from side to side. **Never** nurse head down. Use Fowlers position if possible. Immobile patients need 2 hourly turns.

CHEST INJURIES
EMERGENCY TREATMENT

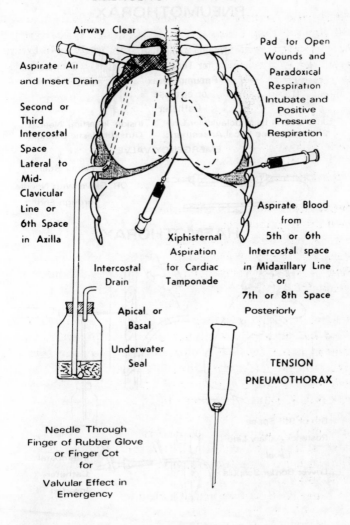

Airway Clear

Aspirate Air
and Insert Drain

Second or
Third
Intercostal
Space
Lateral to
Mid-
Clavicular
Line or
6th Space
in Axilla

Pad for Open
Wounds and
Paradoxical
Respiration

Intubate and
Positive
Pressure
Respiration

Intercostal
Drain

Xiphisternal
Aspiration
for Cardiac
Tamponade

Aspirate Blood
from
5th or 6th
Intercostal space
in Midaxillary Line
or
7th or 8th Space
Posteriorly

Apical or
Basal

Underwater
Seal

TENSION
PNEUMOTHORAX

Needle Through
Finger of Rubber Glove
or Finger Cot
for

Valvular Effect in
Emergency

EMERGENCY RESPIRATION
CHEST ASPIRATION
PNEUMOTHORAX

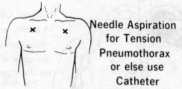

Needle Aspiration
for Tension
Pneumothorax
or else use
Catheter

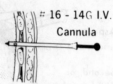

16 - 14G I.V.
Cannula

Just Lateral to Midclavicular Line
2nd Interspace Local Anaesthetic

Inside Inserting Needle
Outside Plastic Cannula

EMERGENCY VALVE

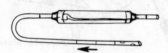

Finger Stall

OR Glove with Needle

Through End

HAEMOTHORAX

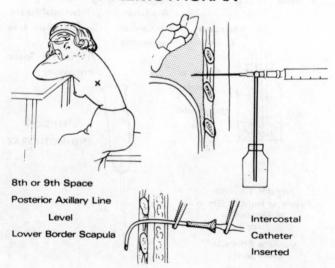

8th or 9th Space
Posterior Axillary Line
Level
Lower Border Scapula

Intercostal
Catheter
Inserted

EMERGENCY TRACHEOSTOMY
ONLY IF INTUBATION IMPOSSIBLE
INSTRUMENTS

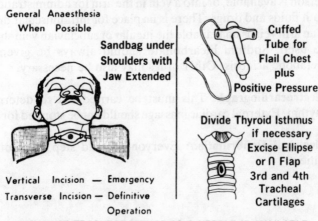

Endotracheal Tube	Tracheal Dilating Forceps	Plastic Tracheo- stomy Tube	Tracheostomy Tube with Removable Inner Cannula	Introducer

FIRST AID - LARGE NEEDLE INTO UPPER TRACHEA

Nasotracheal Intubation in Infants Instead of <u>Tracheostomy</u>

TECHNIQUE

General Anaesthesia
When Possible

**Sandbag under
Shoulders with
Jaw Extended**

**Cuffed
Tube for
Flail Chest
plus
Positive Pressure**

**Divide Thyroid Isthmus
if necessary
Excise Ellipse
or ∩ Flap
3rd and 4th
Tracheal
Cartilages**

Vertical Incision — Emergency
Transverse Incision — Definitive
Operation

ALWAYS USE TRACHEOTOME OR 12 G NEEDLE IF AVAILABLE

CARDIAC ARREST

The most common cause of cardiac arrest is lack of oxygenation of the blood. It is essential therefore, even before cardiac massage is carried out, that the airway is rapidly cleared and the lungs oxygenated by mouth to mouth resuscitation, or by a bag and mask. Immediately after this is done and, without waiting for an endotracheal tube to be passed, the sternum must be compressed according to the illustration with the arms of the resuscitator straight and the hands clenched as illustrated. The legs may be elevated on pillows. The time should be noted and the following should then be carried out.

Intubation of the Patient: This must be carried out by someone skilled in this procedure. Do not attempt intubation before adequate oxygenation if possible.

Intravenous Infusion: Intravenous drip should be inserted as soon as possible, preferably by central catheter, if a skilled person is available, or into a vein in the arm for administration of both fluids and drugs. There is **no** place for intramuscular drugs. If an arm vein is unavailable the jugular or subclavian vein should be used. Sodium bicarbonate should always be given for metabolic acidosis. Other drugs may also be necessary.

Electrocardiograph: This must be carried out to determine rhythm. External cardiac massage should **not** be stopped for this.

Electrical Defibrillation: Everyone should step clear of the patient.

CARDIAC ARREST

Unconscious Apnoea No Carotid Pulse

ACUTE EMERGENCY

START TREATMENT AND

CARDIAC MASSAGE IMMEDIATELY

I V. DRIP
Blood
if
Necessary

Check
Time

CARDIAC
MASSAGE

CLEAR AIRWAY
AND VENTILATE

Check Blood Pressure

Check
Pupils

TREAT CAUSE

Carotid Pulse

ELEVATE FEET

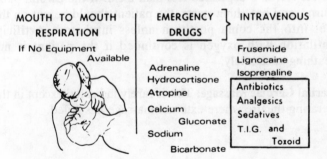

ARTIFICIAL RESPIRATION

MOUTH TO MOUTH RESPIRATION	EMERGENCY DRUGS	INTRAVENOUS
If No Equipment Available	Adrenaline Hydrocortisone Atropine Calcium Gluconate Sodium Bicarbonate	Frusemide Lignocaine Isoprenaline
		Antibiotics Analgesics Sedatives T.I.G. and Toxoid

Pupils & Carotid Pulse: These must be monitored.

Length of Cardiac Massage: This must be carried out for at least three quarters of an hour unless the patient's illness is terminal, such as in secondary carcinomatosis. It is also essential that the underlying cause be rectified as soon as possible. Try intracardiac adrenaline or calcium chloride if all other measures fail, but it is **not** recommended. Intravenous sodium bicarbonate and lignocaine may be necessary.

Method of Cardiac Massage: External massage is carried out, as illustrated, by two clenched interlocked hands over the lower sternum with the elbows straight. The patient should be on a **firm** base such as a solid trolley or floor with the legs elevated. Give cardiac massage **without** delay.

If there are **two operators** there should be one full inflation of the lung to five cardiac compressions, and this should be repeated 12 times per minute. If there is only **one** operator there should be two inflations of the lung to fifteen compressions.

The sternum should be depressed approximately 2 to 4 cm in an adult. In babies two fingers should be used to depress the sternum not more then 1 cm. In children one hand should be used and the sternum depressed less than 2 cm. If the **carotid** pulse returns, and breathing starts, the patient should be put on the side, into the coma postition unless intubated. Artificial ventilation with oxygen is continued if the patient is not breathing adequately.

Internal Cardiac Massage: This is rarely indicated except in the operating theatre where external massage has failed.

CARDIAC ARREST
FURTHER MANAGEMENT

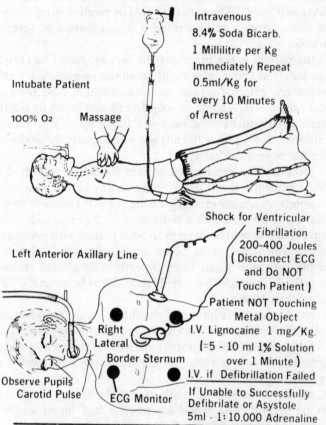

Intravenous
8.4% Soda Bicarb.
1 Millilitre per Kg
Immediately Repeat
0.5ml/Kg for
every 10 Minutes
of Arrest

Intubate Patient

100% O₂   Massage

Shock for Ventricular
Fibrillation
200-400 Joules
(Disconnect ECG
and Do NOT
Touch Patient)

Patient NOT Touching
Metal Object

Left Anterior Axillary Line

I.V. Lignocaine 1 mg/Kg.
(= 5 - 10 ml 1% Solution
over 1 Minute)

Right
Lateral
Border Sternum

I.V. if Defibrillation Failed

Observe Pupils
Carotid Pulse

ECG Monitor

If Unable to Successfully
Defibrilate or Asystole
5ml · 1: 10,000 Adrenaline

Lignocaine Drip 2 - 4 mg min if extrasystoles>6 min
If Defibrillation Fails after Lignocaine give
Adrenaline 0.5mg = 5ml 1:10000 or 0.5ml 1:1000 I.V.
NO INTRACARDIAC DRUGS

DROWNING

If the patient is unconscious and breathing the airway should be cleared of mucus, vomit, dentures and any other debris as quickly as possible. The patient should be positioned on the side in a coma position as illustrated. Oxygen should be given if available.

If the patient is not breathing the airway should be cleared immediately as above, and mouth to mouth resuscitation given. If necessary, external cardiac massage should also be given, as already discussed. An intravenous drip should be set up but the water-logged patient must be given fluids with care. Sodium bicarbonate 8.4% (40 — 100 ml) will be necessary for acidosis if there has been a cardiac arrest.

In hospital the unconscious patient should be intubated as soon as possible, if not maintaining airway or not ventilating adequately. A central venous pressure (C.V.P.) monitor should be set up if possible and a diuretic, such as Frusemide 40mg intravenously should be given to an adult patient with pulmonary oedema which may occur hours after immersion. Pulmonary oedema may well result from hypertonic inhalation and not excess fluid. Therefore Frusemide should only be given if CVP is greater than 10cm.

Steroids may be helpful and should be given intravenously. Antibiotics should also be used to prevent respiratory infection.

A high oxygen intake is important, and the stomach should be emptied as soon as possible as the patient may have swallowed large amounts of water.

Catheterisation and the monitoring of the urinary output may also be helpful. The blood electrolytes and blood levels of oxygen and carbon dioxide should also be assessed.

DROWNING
FIRST AID
PATIENT BREATHING

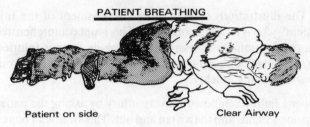

Patient on side   Clear Airway

PATIENT NOT BREATHING

Mouth
to mouth   External Cardiac Massage
Ventilation
After
Clearing Airway

HOSPITAL TREATMENT
UNCONSCIOUS PATIENT

Treat Cerebral and
Pulmonary Oedema
Intubate if Necessary   Lung Complications
Steroids   Cardiac Failure
Antibiotics   Electrolyte Disturbances

HIGH OXYGEN   Empty Stomach
                               Large Bore Tube

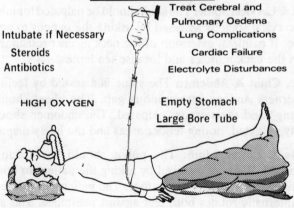

FIRST AID — QUICK ASSESSMENT

The illustrations show a quick "Assessment of the Injured Patient" who is NOT unconscious. This is **not** comprehensive but is a quick 3-minute assessment to exclude serious injuries if a doctor, nurse, ambulance officer or first aider needs to examine several patients quickly.

Upper Limb: Exclude any severe injury by asking the patient to grip one's hands and to twist in and out. This strains all bones and ligaments from the fingers to the shoulder girdle. If the patient has pain the relevant area should be examined in more detail. The pulse should be felt. The median nerve can be tested by abduction of the thumb, the radial nerve by extension of the thumb in the plane of the palm and the ulnar nerve by abduction of the little finger away from the fourth.

Facial Skeleton: Injuries of the orbit and eyes can be seen and the skull palpated. A fracture of the rest of the facial skeleton may be suspected if the patient cannot clench his teeth with the masseters contracting equally.

Head & Cervical Spine: The skull should be palpated for injuries. The cervical spine is assessed by asking the patient to actively rotate. If painless, extension of the neck against resistance will strain the back muscles and localise tenderness.

Spine, Chest & Abdomen The spine is assessed by feeling for tenderness and an interspinous gap. The chest should be "sprung" and the sternum palpated. The abdomen should be briefly palpated, noting tender areas and the likely diagnosis.

Pelvis & Lower Limb: The pelvis should be "sprung" as illustrated. Power is assessed by asking the patient to dorsiflex and plantarflex the big toe or foot. The patient then externally and internally rotates both feet **against** resistance. This strains the entire lower limb from the ankles to the pelvis. Any painful area is then examined.

FIRST AID
QUICK ASSESSMENT
INSPECT PATIENT FOR OBVIOUS INJURIES AND SHOCK
UPPER LIMBS

Assess -
- Power
- Major Fracture or Dislocation
- Circulation

Pulse
- Circulation
- Shock

GRIP Examiners Hand

Twist In

Twist out

FACIAL SKELETON AND SKULL

ORBIT AND EYES - Inspect

NOSE - Inspect and Palpate

CLENCH TEETH - Equal contraction

of masseters means   NO <u>Serious</u>

Mandibular or Maxillary Damage

(<u>Except</u> orbit and nose)

CERVICAL SPINE

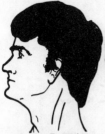

Active Rotation to right

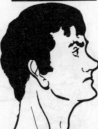

Active Rotation to left

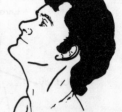

Extend Against Resistance

IF PAINLESS - Eliminates likelihood of severe Injury

FIRST AID
QUICK ASSESSMENT

SPINE

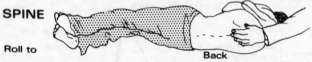

Roll to
Opposite Side

Back
Interspinous Gap
Palpate Supraspinous Processes
Other Tenderness

CHEST

Respiratory
Distress or Difficulty

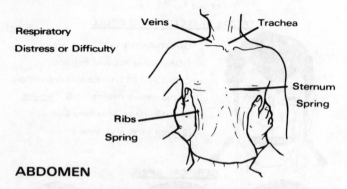

Veins

Trachea

Sternum
Spring

Ribs
Spring

ABDOMEN

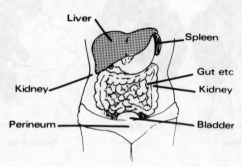

Liver

Spleen

Gut etc

Kidney

Kidney

Perineum

Bladder

FIRST AID
QUICK ASSESSMENT
PELVIS

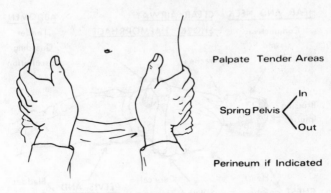

Palpate Tender Areas

Spring Pelvis $\Big\langle$ In / Out

Perineum if Indicated

LOWER LIMBS

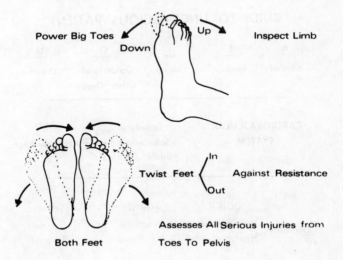

Power Big Toes — Up — Inspect Limb
Down

Twist Feet $\Big\langle$ In / Out — Against Resistance

Both Feet

Assesses All Serious Injuries from Toes To Pelvis

EXAMINATION IN MAJOR TRAUMA
HISTORY AND EXAMINATION

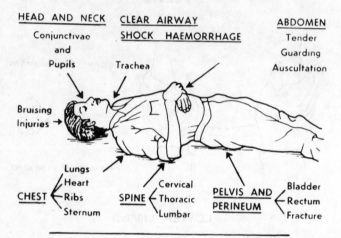

HEAD AND NECK
Conjunctivae
and
Pupils

CLEAR AIRWAY
SHOCK HAEMORRHAGE

ABDOMEN
Tender
Guarding
Auscultation

Trachea

Bruising
Injuries →

CHEST ←
Lungs
Heart
Ribs
Sternum

SPINE ←
Cervical
Thoracic
Lumbar

PELVIS AND
PERINEUM ←
Bladder
Rectum
Fracture

GUIDE TO UNCONSCIOUS PATIENT

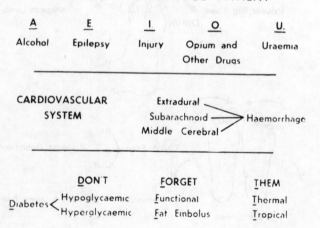

A	**E**	**I**	**O**	**U.**
Alcohol	Epilepsy	Injury	Opium and Other Drugs	Uraemia

CARDIOVASCULAR
SYSTEM

Extradural
Subarachnoid ——→ Haemorrhage
Middle Cerebral

DON'T	**F**ORGET	**T**HEM
Diabetes < **H**ypoglycaemic / **H**yperglycaemic	**F**unctional / **F**at Embolus	**T**hermal / **T**ropical

EXAMINATION

UPPER AND LOWER LIMBS

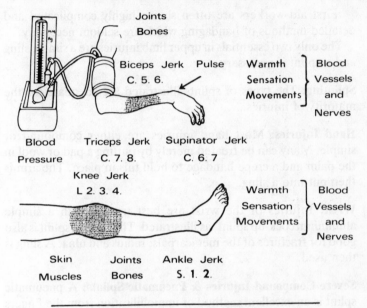

Joints
Bones

Biceps Jerk   Pulse   Warmth   Blood
C. 5. 6.   Sensation   Vessels
                Movements   and

                             Nerves

Blood   Triceps Jerk   Supinator Jerk

Pressure   C. 7. 8.   C. 6. 7.

Knee Jerk

L 2. 3. 4.   Warmth   Blood
                          Sensation   Vessels
                          Movements   and

                             Nerves

Skin   Joints   Ankle Jerk

Muscles   Bones   S. 1. 2.

GUIDE TO REFLEXES

1
2 } S — Ankle Jerk   Supinator Jerk C. 6. 7.

3
4 } L — Knee Jerk   B before T in alphabet

5
6 } C — Biceps Jerk   B. J. C. 5 6 before

7
8 } C — Triceps Jerk   T. J. C. 7. 8

FIRST AID — SPLINTING OF UPPER LIMB

First aid workers are often shown highly complicated and detailed methods of bandaging which are seldom necessary.

The only two essentials in upper limb injuries are a simple sling and a splint if necessary.

Splinting: The types of splints illustrated are adequate for the majority of injuries.

Hand Injuries: Most hand injuries are either compound or simple. Many can be treated merely by putting a pad of wool in the palm and a crepe bandage to hold this in place. The arm is then put into a sling.

Wrist: Injuries of the wrist are best treated with a simple aluminium cock-up splint, as illustrated. This type of splint is also good for fractures of the metacarpals, radius and ulna. A sling is then used.

Severe Compound Injuries & Pneumatic Splints: A pneumatic splint is an excellent method of immobilisation from the fingers to the lower humerus.

It has the advantage that the wound can be seen, and x-rays can be carried out **without** removing the splint. This type of splint is particularly useful in compound fractures which are bleeding and which need pressure. It can be used for severe fractures of the arm or the leg, before x-ray of the patient in hospital. It will save shock and excessive movement of the limb. Dangers include the increase of relative pressure when a patient is travelling by car or aeroplane at a height of over 1,000 metres, and increase in pressure in the hot sun. The splint should only be inflated by mouth and **not** by a pump.

EMERGENCY SPLINTING
UPPER LIMB
ALL SEVERE HAND INJURIES

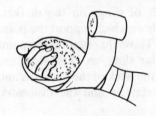

Hand Bandaged Over Wool Sling

FRACTURES AROUND WRIST

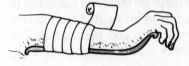

Aluminium Cock Up Splint

Note
Right
Left
Splints

ALL SEVERE INJURIES FINGER TO LOWER HUMERUS

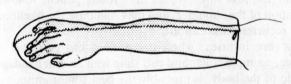

Pneumatic Splint NOT by Air over 1000 metres

TEMPORARY SPLINT

If no splint is available one can be made from a rolled newspaper or wood covered with cloth. The limb is then bandaged to this. A splint can also be made out of plaster of Paris. The arm should then be put in a triangular sling. In major injuries the limb is bandaged to the side of the body.

UPPER LIMB SLING

There are many different kinds of slings on the market. Basically they can be divided into those which support the point of the elbow and those that do not. Those that support the point of the elbow such as the **triangular** sling, as illustrated, are **absolutely** indicated in fractures of the neck of the humerus and the shoulder girdle, such as the clavicle and the dislocated acromio-clavicular joint.

Those that do not support the point of the elbow are the simple collar and cuff slings and these are indicated **absolutely** in only one condition. This is a fracture of the **shaft** of the humerus as this allows the weight of the arm to pull the fracture into alignment. In all other cases either type of sling can be used, depending on availability.

In a dislocation of the shoulder, after reduction, a double type of collar and cuff, as illustrated, is the coolest and best and this prevents the arm from rotating externally. This is sometimes used for the first three weeks in a young patient following a dislocation of the shoulder, and may minimise the likelihood of future recurrent dislocation.

In severe injuries, when the patient has to travel some distance, a simple collar and cuff sling with an arm bandaged to the side of the body, is probably the best compromise.

UPPER LIMB SLINGS

TRIANGULAR SLING

DOUBLE COLLAR AND CUFF

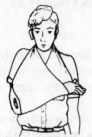

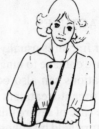

All Injuries Except Shaft Humerus

COLLAR AND CUFF

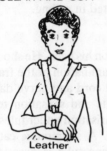

Wool

Around Wrist

and

Behind Neck

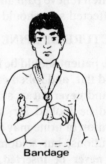

Leather

Bandage

NOT for Fractures Clavicle Neck Humerus and

Dislocation Acromio— Clavicular Joint

COLLAR AND CUFF WITH ARM TO SIDE

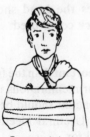

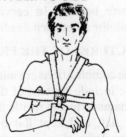

Severe Injuries

Dislocation Shoulder After Reduction

FRACTURE OF TRUNK
EMERGENCY TREATMENT

RIB FRACTURES

Minor fractures usually require no treatment. Major fractures may cause damage to lung, heart or abdominal viscera, and these complications can also occur with minor rib fractures and will require urgent treatment.

In the case of **severe** unstable rib fractures, a pad of wool over the fracture held by adhesive strapping or an encircling bandage, will often relieve pain and help the patient to cough. The arm on the affected side should always be rested in a sling.

FRACTURE OF SPINE

The patient should be kept flat lying on his back. He should be moved flat, and rolled carefully for examination of the fracture site, and **never** sat or stood up. Spinal cord and nerve damage should be looked for, and movements and sensation tested. Retention of urine may require catheterisation under full sterile precautions, but seldom immediately. A suprapubic catheter must **never be inserted,** fine polythene tube is occasionally indicated. If no stretcher is available, the patient should be carried face down, with the spine hyperextended. **Never** let the spine flex. In hospital, the patient should be on a mattress on fracture boards. In cervical fractures the head should be immobilised between sandbags or a neck collar used.

FRACTURES OF THE PELVIS

The complications are much more important than the fracture. These include rupture of the bladder or membranous urethra, and damage to the sciatic nerve. The patient should be moved lying flat, and kept flat on his back. Urethral bleeding and extravasation of urine must be watched for.

EMERGENCY SPLINTING TRUNK
CERVICAL SPINE

Simple Neck Collar

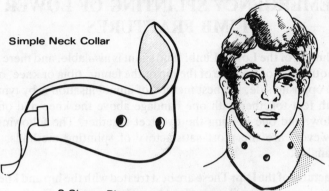

3 Sizes - Plastazote with Velcro Fastening

THORACIC AND LUMBAR SPINE

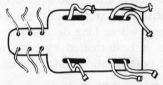

Spinal

Board

Transport of Patients with Spinal Injuries

EMERGENCY STRETCHER

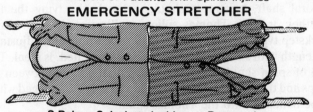

2 Poles - 2 Jackets Inside out Buttoned up

N.B. Transport Patients

with Thoracic and Lumbar Spinal Injuries

Face Down if No Stretchers Available

EMERGENCY SPLINTING OF LOWER LIMB FRACTURES

Splinting of the Lower Limb: If no splint is available, and there is no other major fracture of the hip or the femur, tibia or knee, on the opposite side, the best method of immobilisation is by tying both feet together with one bandage above the knee and one below, and one holding the two feet together. The following, however, are the most satisfactory of splinting methods, if available.

Fractures of the Hip: These are best treated with the hip and knee flexed over 2 or 3 pillows and **not** by a Thomas splint. The flexion will correct the usual external rotation of a hip fracture. This treatment is also used in hospital as a pre-operative method. It is also the most satisfactory treatment at present for travelling by ambulance, except where long distances are involved. In this case the patient is best treated by tying both legs and feet together to hold both rotation and alignment.

Fractures of the Femoral Shaft: In fractures of the mid or lower femoral shaft, treatment should either be by tying the feet together or by a Thomas splint, as illustrated. A modified Huckstep type Thomas splint with an open ring, and adjustable for length with straps behind the leg, as illustrated, is ideal. This type of splint should be padded with plaster wool between the straps and the leg. The leg should then be lightly bandaged with a crepe bandage onto the Thomas splint.

If the patient is to be transported a long distance and if skin traction is available, this should be applied as shown. It is important that, when traction is used, the foot is inspected regularly to make sure that the traction is not constricting the blood supply to the foot.

In patients travelling long distances plaster of Paris or crepe bandages over wool to hold the whole leg into the Thomas splint should be used. If plaster is used it is essential that this be split before the patient is transported.

HIP FRACTURES
EMERGENCY TREATMENT

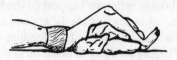

Correct
External
Rotation

Leg Flexed
Over 2-3 Pillows
or Bandage Legs
Together

Do NOT Use Thomas Splint

OPEN FRACTURES AND INJURIES

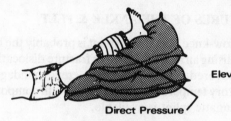

Elevation

Direct Pressure

Over Large Pad of Wool

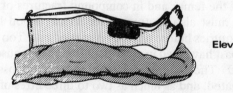

Elevation

Pneumatic Splint Over Large Pad
NOT BY AIR OVER 1000 METRES

NOTE Direct Pressure **NOT** Tourniquet in Nearly **All** Cases

FRACTURES OF THE KNEE & TIBIA

The emergency treatment of these fractures is to bandage the leg to a Thomas splint. If necessary traction can also be used. An alternative to a Thomas splint for support of the **lower** femur, as well as the knee, tibia and ankle is a pneumatic splint. A pneumatic splint is also invaluable for bleeding or for splinting the leg in hospital before an x-ray. If no splint is available the legs should be tied together, as with the femur.

If both legs are fractured, splinting can be carried out by using a piece of wood padded with cloth or by using rolled up newspaper as a longitudinal support.

FRACTURES OF THE ANKLE & FEET

A below-knee pneumatic splint is probably the best method of immobilising an ankle fracture or fracture dislocation. A wooden splint covered with wool and a crepe bandage is the most satisfactory **temporary** measure, even with compound injuries, if no pneumatic splint is available.

The lower limb should be elevated to reduce oedema in **all** severe fractures of the lower limb. This is particularly so for the shaft of the femur and in compound fractures of the tibia. The patient must also be treated for shock, blood loss and other major injuries before an x-ray is carried out. Too many patients in the past have died in x-ray departments because this has been omitted. The extent of shock and blood loss is often not appreciated, and as much as two to three litres of blood may be lost in fractures of the femoral shafts.

EMERGENCY SPLINTING LOWER LIMB

OPPOSITE LEG

3 Bandages

Above Knee   Below Knee   Feet Together

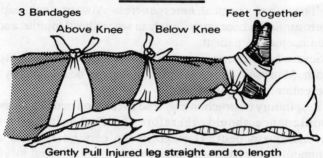

Gently Pull Injured leg straight and to length

THOMAS SPLINT (Huckstep Modification)

Adjustable Top

Adjustable for Length

Single Splint Left or Right

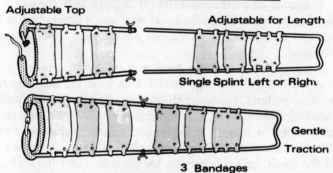

Gentle Traction

3 Bandages

PNEUMATIC SPLINT

Useful for Bleeding

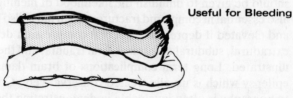

Lower Femur to Toes

NOT BY AIR OVER 1000 METRES

HEAD INJURIES

These are surgical emergencies. Always seek expert neurosurgical advice immediately in severe head injuries and in the unconscious patient.

Severe head injuries may lead to severe residual disability or death. Many side effects of head injuries can be lessened by the prevention of complications.

Respiratory obstruction may lead to cerebral oedema. Airway maintenance should, therefore, be **first** priority in the unconscious patient. Damage to the cervical spine is also commonly associated with head injuries, and a lateral x-ray of the cervical spine is essential in **all** unconscious patients.

Evidence of increasing cerebral compression consists of a slowing pulse, a rising blood pressure, and a diminution of the level of consciousness. A careful neurological examination is essential.

Damage to the **anterior fossa** may be deduced by posterior conjunctival haemorrhage or CSF leak from the nose together with, or without, epistaxis. **Middle fossa** damage is suggested by bleeding from the ear, it is confirmed by CSF leak, and rarely announced by **seventh or eighth** nerve damage. **Posterior fossa** damage should be considered with either bleeding from the back of the throat or a suboccipital haematoma under the scalp.

In fractures of the anterior and middle fossa, chemotherapy should be given to diminish the likelihood of meningitis. This is also essential in compound fractures which must also be explored and elevated if depressed. Cerebral compression develops with extradural, subdural or intracerebral trauma, and these signs are illustrated. Long term complications of brain damage include epilepsy which is usually treated conservatively. Computerised tomography is often invaluable in demonstrating the formation of a haematoma, localised cerebral pressure by clot, fluid or oedema.

Brain scan with a radioisotope may also show localised areas if there is uptake in damaged areas, but is rarely used.

HEAD INJURIES
EXAMINATION
GENERAL

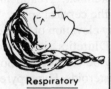

Slowing Pulse
Rising Systolic B.P.
Neurological Signs
Deterioration Level
Consciousness

| Respiratory Obstruction | Cervical Spine Other Injuries | Cerebral Compression |

LOCAL

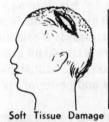

Anterior
Middle ⟶ Fossa
Posterior

| Soft Tissue Damage | Fracture Vault | Fracture Base |

Haematoma

NEUROLOGICAL

Size Pupils + Reaction
Dilated Side
of
Lesion

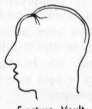

Papilloedema

Movement and
Tone
Sensation
Reflexes

State of
Consciousness
Alert.
Drowsy.
Stuporous.
Comatose

CSF

Fundi

1–2 HOURLY CHECK ON PATIENT

All patients with head injuries must be carefully examined for spinal injuries and injuries of the limbs, trunk and abdomen.

Non-surgical treatment of head injuries should include keeping the airway clear, preventing bed sores and contractures of limbs, and management of urinary retention. Treatment of associated injuries includes fractures of the cervical spine.

The treatment of cerebral oedema is by elevation of the head of the bed, and restriction of fluids. Diuretics, intravenous mannitol and triple strength plasma may be considered. Some surgeons used to advise the use of corticosteroids. Hyperpyrexia is best treated by cooling with a fan or air-conditioner. Localised cerebral compression must also be looked for on evidence of neurological deficit. Anti-convulsants may be indicated for convulsions.

In the case of cerebral compression by haematoma, if investigations such as C.T. scanning are not available, the brain should be inspected by burr holes, as illustrated. It is essential that both sides of the skull be drilled if there is any doubt about compression on the opposite side. In addition it is essential that, in most cases, burr holes be **both** anterior and posterior, as a localised haematoma is possible.

The long-term management of the patient may be difficult and this consists mainly of nursing with catheterisation if necessary, aspiration of pharynx and the prevention of respiratory obstruction. Two-hourly turning day and night is important for the care of the skin and the prevention of joint contractures. The feeding of unconscious patients is best done by a naso-gastric tube but intravenous fluids may be necessary. Drugs may be needed for restlessness (chlorpromazine), and to prevent both bladder and respiratory infections (antibiotics). Long-term management will include rehabilitation, preferably in a special centre and anticonvulsants for epilepsy. There is only a very occasional place for surgery in epilepsy, due to depressed skull or scarring of the meninges.

HEAD INJURIES
CEREBRAL DAMAGE

Reticular Formation
Affected

head trauma

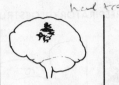

| Concussion | Contusion | Cerebral Laceration |

CEREBRAL COMPRESSION

Haemorrhages

	Venous	Oedema or Blood Clot
Unilateral	Older Patient	May Affect
Early Signs	Early or Late	Basal Centres
Young Patient	Signs	Early Marked Signs
Lucid Interval		
Extradural	**Subdural**	**Intracerebral**

WITH OR WITHOUT FRACTURE

BASAL FRACTURES

Posterior
Conjunctival
Haemorrhage

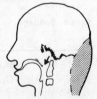

C. S. F. Leak	Bleeding Ear	Bleeding Back
Nose	C.S.F. **Leak**	of Throat
Epistaxis	7th and 8th	Suboccipital Bleeding
	Nerve Damage	
Anterior Fossa	**Middle Fossa**	**Posterior Fossa**

DANGER OF MENINGITIS

HEAD INJURIES
EMERGENCY TREATMENT
RESPIRATORY OBSTRUCTION

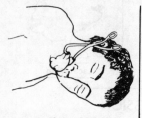 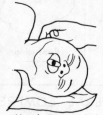 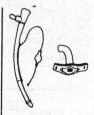

Clear Airway	Head Down and To Side Oral Airway	Intubate or Tracheostomy If Necessary

OPEN WOUNDS	CEREBRAL OEDEMA

OPEN WOUNDS

Inspect for F.B.'s
and Fractures
X—ray
Chemotherapy
Suture
Crepe Bandage

CEREBRAL OEDEMA

Restrict Fluids Give Diuretics
Steroids Special Cases Only

ELEVATE HEAD
Cool Patient if Pyrexia
Exposure, Fan or Cold Sponging

30% Mannitol ⎫
3X Strength ⎬ I.V.
Plasma   ⎭

BRAIN COMPRESSION
Operate If in Doubt

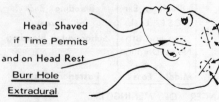

Head Shaved
if Time Permits
and on Head Rest
Burr Hole
Extradural

Skin Incisions
and
Burr Holes
Subdural

ALWAYS INSPECT BOTH SIDES IF NECESSARY

HEAD INJURIES

NURSING

HEAD MUST BE ELEVATED
Aspiration of Pharynx   Catheter if
Necessary

2 Hourly ⎫ Day and
Turning ⎭ night

CARE ⟨ Skin
       Joints
       Bladder

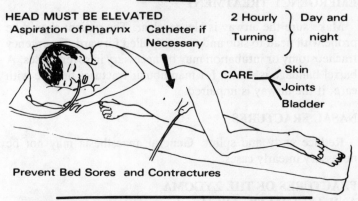

Prevent Bed Sores and Contractures

RESPIRATORY INFECTION

Breathing Exercises
and
Chemotherapy
Orotracheal Tube
if Necessary
in Early Stages

FEEDING AND FLUIDS

Gastric Tube if Cannot Swallow
OR

I.V. FLUIDS

ADULT ⟨ 24hrs – NIL
        24hrs – 500ml
        24hrs – 1,000ml

BLADDER AND BOWELS

Catheter — Avoid Infection
Penrose Tube Later
Prevent — Faecal Impaction

NEVER MORPHIA
ASPIRIN FOR PAIN
CHLORPROMAZINE IF RESTLESS

REHABILITATION

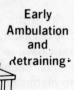

Early
Ambulation
and
Retraining

FACE AND JAW INJURIES

EMERGENCY TREATMENT

Make sure the airway is always clear. The patient should be prone with head to side and tongue pulled forward. Emergency tracheostomy or intubation may be necessary in severe cases. A barrel bandage is shown for mandibular fractures but use with care, if the airway is impaired.

NASAL FRACTURES

Reduce early and splint. General anaesthesia may not be necessary in early cases.

FRACTURES OF THE ZYGOMA AND ZYGOMATIC ARCH

Elevate with retractor inserted above hairline on side of depression. Watch for diplopia.

FRACTURES OF THE MANDIBLE

Diagnosis:

History of trauma
Pain and swelling at site
Patient complaining of teeth not occluding

Radiographs:

Panoramic (OPG) of mandible
PA of mandible

Splinting of the teeth is required in most cases with displacement, presuming that the maxilla is sound. The patient must have most of his natural teeth for eyelet wire or arch-bar splints. Edentulous patients **must** keep their dentures with them, no matter how badly broken, as this makes the best splint. All parts of broken dentures must be accounted for as denture material is radiolucent. Call the dentist early if the denture is to be adapted or a Gunning splint made for an edentulous patient. A barrel bandage is of use only for a bilateral fracture with displacement.

FACE AND JAW INJURIES
MAXILLA

EMERGENCY TREATMENT
KEEP AIRWAY CLEAR

Prone Head to Side	Tongue Pulled Forward	Tracheostomy if Necessary	Remove Broken Teeth or Dentures from Mouth

Disimpact if Necessary

Cranio-Mandibular Fixation

4—5 Weeks   Traction or Refracture may be Required

Orbital Floor May be Depressed

Expert Advice Essential

Elevate Depressed Zygoma if Necessary

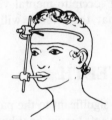

TEETH

BROKEN TOOTH	LOOSENED OR DISPLACED TOOTH	COMPLETELY DISPLACED TOOTH

See Dentist Quickly To Avoid Discoloration	Push Back in into Place See Dentist for Splinting	Replace in Socket Keep Moist with Warm Saline See Dentist for Splinting

FRACTURE OF THE MAXILLA

Displacement is usually downwards and backwards threatening the airway. Reduction will require skilled treatment with splints and cranial fixation. Check that the airway is clear and that bleeding has stopped. Patient must be kept under close observation. Aspirate regularly. Intubation is indicated instead of tracheostomy where this is possible. Notify dentist early as splint production takes time.

Radiographs True lateral, 10° and 30° occipito-mental views. Conscious patients will complain that their teeth will not occlude; this is diagnostic.

INJURIES TO TEETH

Injuries to the teeth are often more significant to the patient than laceration of the soft tissues. The soft tissues heal but the teeth remain broken and discolour. Consultation with the dentist is a matter of urgency if the patient is to be treated properly.

FRACTURED TEETH

Broken teeth and even teeth bumped and not broken, need urgent dental attention if they are not to discolour.

DISPLACED TEETH

Whether totally or partially displaced these should be gently, but firmly, pushed back into the socket. The dentist should be urgently consulted for splinting and endodontic therapy. Totally displaced teeth should be kept in gauze soaked in warm saline if not replanted until replantation can be carried out.

FACE AND JAW INJURIES

MANDIBLE

TREATMENT

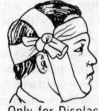

Clear Airway

Emergency
Bandage

Only for Displaced Fractures of the Mandible

Interdental Eyelet Wiring

Against

Sound Maxillary Arch

DENTURES & JAW FRACTURES

Dentures Even when Badly Broken Should be Kept

with the Patient

Dentures often Make the Best Splints

POST OPERATIVE

Sedate	Fluids	1/4 – 1/2
Anti Emetic	Only by Mouth	Hourly Check
Aspiration	Antibiotics	Respiration
Mucus	Mouth Wash	Cut Wires in
		Emergency and
		Laryngoscope

MOUTH AND THROAT EMERGENCIES

Mouth and throat emergencies cause considerable distress, often out of all proportion to their seriousness.

A cut or bitten tongue is common and will bleed considerably. These heal well, except when very large, and do not usually require sutures. In any case this should be done with absorbable sutures. Antibiotics are seldom necessary.

A fish bone in the throat or larynx is a surgical emergency, and if not seen by indirect laryngoscopy the patient should be x-rayed. A small piece of cotton wool impregnated with barium if swallowed may catch on the bone and show the position on x-ray.

Laryngeal foreign bodies are common in children and these are surgical emergencies. The patient must **always** be admitted to hospital. Foreign bodies such as peanuts may not be seen on x-ray. The peanut may act as a valve causing over-inflation and thus radiolucency of the lung on the **obstructed** side. The patient may also need to be bronchoscoped. Fractures of the nose, if causing deformity, will need reduction **irrespective** of appearance of the x-ray. The same will apply to septal deviation. A septal haematoma will require drainage on both sides and antibiotics.

A severe epistaxis may require packing with Vaseline gauze. Occasionally 4 ml of 4% Lignocaine and 0.5 ml, 1/1000 adrenaline for 5 minutes is indicated.

Foreign bodies in the ear are common, particularly in children, and may require removal with correct instruments in an Ear, Nose and Throat department. Insects may be attracted out of the ear with a bright light. If not they should be killed with spirit before removing. Whisky or gin can also be used in an emergency!

Perforations of the tympanic membrane should be treated with antibiotics and referred to an Ear, Nose and Throat specialist **without** removing clot and wax, and **without** syringing the ear or inserting ear drops.

MOUTH AND THROAT EMERGENCIES

CUT OR BITTEN TONGUE

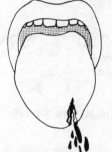

Suture Only Large Lacerations

2% Xylocaine with

Adrenaline + Absorbable Suture

Mouth washes

Antibiotics - Rarely Needed

FISH BONES - THROAT OR LARYNX

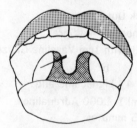

Inspect Tonsils

Indirect Laryngoscopy

X-Ray if Negative -

(Barium and Cotton Wool)

SWALLOWED OR INHALED FOREIGN BODY

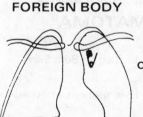

X-RAY CHEST ⟨ A.P. / LATERAL

Oesophagoscope or Bronchoscope if necessary

SURGICAL EMERGENCY
ADMIT PATIENT

CRUSHED LARYNX – MAY REQUIRE INTUBATION

INJURIES TO NOSE
FRACTURED NOSE

Manipulation within
5 Days of Accident

Suture Lacerations
Over Fracture

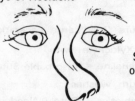

Small Plaster
of Paris Mould
Strap On

DEFORMITY ALWAYS NEEDS REDUCTION WITHIN 5 DAYS
IRRESPECTIVE OF X-RAY

EPISTAXIS

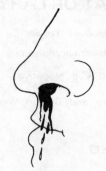

Suck Out Blood
Lignocaine 4% Spray
Pack with 1cm Vaseline Gauze
or
4ml 4% Lignocaine and
0.5ml 1/1,000 Adrenaline
for 5 minutes

Cauterize if Necessary

SEPTAL HAEMATOMA

Always Needs Incision on Both Sides

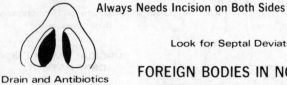

Look for Septal Deviation

Drain and Antibiotics

FOREIGN BODIES IN NOSE
SEEK EXPERT ATTENTION

EAR INJURIES

FOREIGN BODIES

BEADS AND STONES

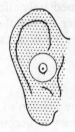

Remove with Proper Instruments
(**Not** Forceps)
Never Attempt to Remove Hard Foreign
Bodies Send Patient to Ear/Nose/Throat
(E.N.T.) Surgeon if Possible

INSECTS

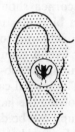

Kill with Any Kind of Spirit
Even Whisky or Gin

Remove Carefully

PERFORATION OF TYMPANIC MEMBRANE

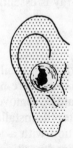

Remove Clot or Wax

DO **NOT** — Syringe

Insert Ear Drops

COTTON WOOL IN OUTER EAR
COMMENCE ANTIBIOTICS
REFER TO E.N.T. SPECIALIST

EYE INJURIES

HISTORY

An adequate history is essential, and this will include details of the injury and whether visual acuity was immediately affected. The history of use of power tools, a hammer on metal or an explosion may require an x-ray of the orbit to exclude a retained orbital or intraocular foreign body.

EXAMINATION

Visual acuity should be estimated using the Snellen's Chart. Local anaesthetic such as 0.5% amethocaine may be necessary if the patient cannot open the eyelids and after this the eye should always be padded. The conjunctiva and cornea should be inspected with magnification such as with a binocular loupe. Fluorescein is instilled in the lower conjunctional fornix to stain any corneal epithelial defects. The upper eyelid should be everted to look for superficial foreign bodies along the sub-tarsal fold and in the upper conjunctival fornix. The medial canthal area should be inspected for lacerations involving the lacrimal system. If a retinal lesion is suspected the pupil can be dilated with a short acting mydriatic such as 0.5% Mydriacyl.

Fractures of the orbital bones may cause enophthalmos and vertical diplopia due to trapping of the inferior rectus muscle with limitation of elevation of the eye. An x-ray is essential to show the sinuses and orbital floor.

TREATMENT OF EYE INJURIES

Minor foreign bodies on the conjunctiva may easily be removed with a cotton wool pledget but with great care not to abraid the cornea. Corneal foreign bodies should be removed by a sharp instrument such as a 21 gauge needle after the installation of a local anaesthetic. If possible, magnification with a loupe should be used with the patient's head in a fixed position in a chair or couch.

EYE INJURIES
EXAMINATION

HISTORY

Eliminate other causes with similar symptoms

DIRECT INSPECTION

Evert Upper Eyelid

Fluorescein

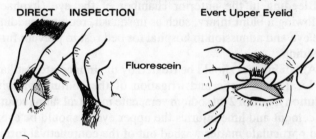

OPHTHALMOSCOPE

Sclera

cornea

(<u>Never</u> Atropine)

Care Shallow

Anterior Chamber)

AFTER

EXAMINATION

Always Pad

after Local Anaesthetic

MAGNIFYING GLASS

Short Acting Mydriatics
such as Tropicamide

0.5 % Mydriacyl

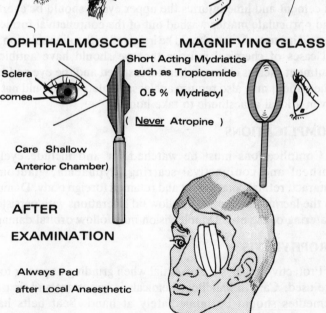

Patients with possible retained intraocular foreign bodies or penetrating injuries should have the eye padded, an antibiotic drop instilled and be admitted to hospital under the care of an ophthalmic surgeon. X-ray will confirm the presence of a retained foreign body in the orbit or eye.

Bleeding in the anterior chamber of the eye (hyphaema) following a blunt injury, such as in squash, requires padding of the eye and admission to hospital for bed rest to prevent further bleeding.

Alkali injuries should be treated by the **immediate** instillation of local anaesthetic and irrigation of the conjunctiva with a solution made of 2 ml sodium versenate in 100 ml saline solution. In cement and lime injuries the upper eyelid should be everted and particulate matter washed out of the conjunctival fornices. In acid injuries the eye should be irrigated with saline solution. In all cases of chemical injuries the eye should have antibiotic ointment such as chloramphenicol instilled and the eye padded. The patient may also require analgesic tablets but should **not** be given a local anaesthetic to take home.

COMPLICATIONS

Complications must be watched for and include eyelid, corneal and conjunctival scarring, hyphaema, glaucoma, cataract, retinal detachment and retained foreign body. Damage to the lacrimal system may follow lid lacerations with persistent watering of the eye. Double vision may follow orbital damage.

PROPHYLAXIS

Protective goggles are essential when grinding or power tools are used. Care in handling chemicals is important and first aid remedies should be immediately at hand. Seat belts have lowered the incidence of windscreen injuries. First aid workers must perform early treatment. Early treatment in all eye injuries and education in emergency care is essential.

EYE INJURIES
CORNEAL FOREIGN BODIES

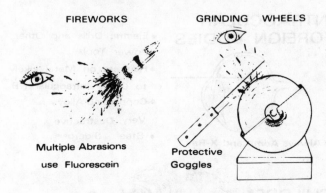

FIREWORKS

Multiple Abrasions
use Fluorescein

GRINDING WHEELS

Protective
Goggles

REMOVAL

Chair with Head Rest
or Lie Patient on Couch

Use
Magnification

Amethocaine ½%

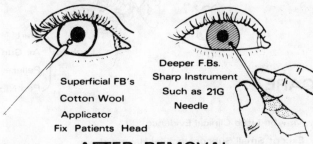

Superficial FB's
Cotton Wool
Applicator
Fix Patients Head

Deeper F.Bs.
Sharp Instrument
Such as 21G
Needle

AFTER REMOVAL

Local

Antibiotics-

Eye Pad

CARE - DO NOT Mistake Scleral Perforating Vessels
with Subconjunctival Pigment for Foreign Bodies

EYE INJURIES
PERFORATING INJURIES

INTRAOCULAR FOREIGN BODIES

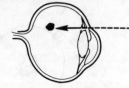

- Electric Drills and Other Power Tools
- Hammer on Metal Likely to Cause Intraocular F.B.
- Copper and Alloys Very Destructive
- Steel Siderosis

Always Admit and X-Ray

CHILDREN

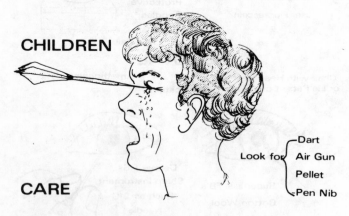

Look for
- Dart
- Air Gun
- Pellet
- Pen Nib

CARE

May be Little Clinical Evidence
Except Small Subconjunctival Haemorrhage

SCISSORS AND WINDSCREEN
IRREGULAR PUPIL

Antibiotics   Pad
Admit and Refer to Eye Surgeon

EYE INJURIES
BLUNT INJURIES

Squash Injury

HYPHAEMA

Fist

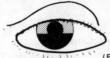

Early
or
Late

Admit

Bilateral Eye Pads

(5 - 7 days)

LENS SUBLUXATION

DETACHED RETINA

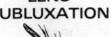

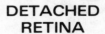

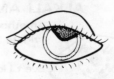

Admit

Admit

Flashes of Light

Floaters

Shadow

FRACTURE OF ORBITAL BONES

Enophthalmos

Look for Bruising Lids

Xray - May NOT
always
Show Fracture

Blow out Fracture
through Orbital Floor

Surgical Crepitus
(Fracture into sinus)

Defective Elevation Eye = Inferior Rectus Trapped
by Orbital Fat

EYE
CHEMICAL AND THERMAL BURNS

ACIDS

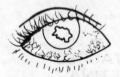

Irrigate Immediately

with SALINE

ALKALI AND LIME BURNS

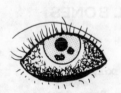

Amethocaine

Irrigate Immediately - 2ml. Sodium Versenate
in 100ml. Saline

Evert Lids and Remove Lime from Fornices

Conjunctival Adhesions May Occur

FLASH KERATITIS

Severe Ocular Irritation

Watering Several Hours Later

Amethocaine + Fluorescein

Numerous Small Stained AREAS

Recovers Within 24hours

ANTIBIOTICS   ANALGESIA   EYE PAD

EYE INJURIES
COMPLICATIONS

BLUNT INJURIES

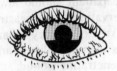

HYPHAEMA Early

Treat Early Late

CATARACT

VITREOUS HAEMORRHAGE

DETACHED RETINA

LID LACERATION

Damage to Inner Canthus
Lacrimal Canaliculi May Be
Damaged EPIPHORA

STRABISMUS
OR
ENOPHTHALMOS

DISTORTION CORNEA
DUE TO SCARRING

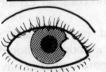

Prevent Infection

Refraction
May Need Corneal Graft

RUST STAINING
CORNEA

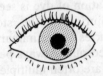

Remove Foreign Bodies Early

ABDOMINAL INJURIES

Always consider all the organs likely to be damaged in a closed or open injury of the abdomen. If there is any doubt whatsoever of visceral damage the patient should always be admitted to hospital for careful observation. A nasogastric tube should be immediately inserted. An exploratory laparotomy must **always** be carried out if there is any possibility of an injury involving the gut, spleen and in all penetrating wounds, and also if there is any evidence of bleeding or peritonitis. Always perform a rectal examination and auscultate the abdomen in **all cases,** and always carry out a full examination of the urine including the presence of blood, as well as serum amylase in blunt trauma to exclude pancreatic damage.

Spleen: This may be ruptured by minimal violence, especially if enlarged due to disease. A lower posterior rib fracture is particularly liable to damage the spleen. Local tenderness in the left hypochondrium, pain referred to the left shoulder, dullness in the flanks which may not shift on the left, a rising pulse rate, increasing anaemia and dyspnoea are all valuable signs which may **not** always be present. Always perform a laparotomy if in doubt, and perform a splenectomy or repair.

Liver: Injuries to the liver, if **minor,** can be treated conservatively. Gall bladder injuries, however, require exploration and excision or drainage in all cases.

Kidney: Renal injuries are usually treated **conservatively** unless major. **Always** perform an intravenous pyelogram to ensure that the opposite kidney is functioning and consider exploration if extravasation of dye is seen.

Gut: Injuries of the stomach and intestines are surgical emergencies. A preliminary x-ray of the abdomen should always be carried out. Always perform a laparotomy if in any doubt. Injuries are often multiple and the entire gut must be carefully inspected. The mesentery may also be damaged. Small intestine of doubtful viability must always be resected. Damaged large intestine will require a colostomy.

ABDOMINAL INJURIES

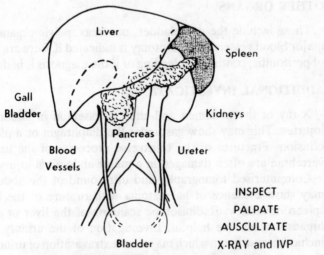

Liver

Spleen

Gall Bladder

Kidneys

Pancreas

Blood Vessels

Ureter

INSPECT
PALPATE
AUSCULTATE
X-RAY and IVP

Bladder

CT SCAN and ULTRASOUND FOR LIVER. SPLEEN
and KIDNEY DAMAGE IF NECESSARY

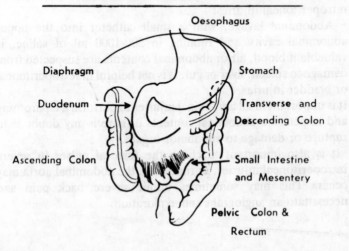

Oesophagus

Diaphragm

Stomach

Duodenum

Transverse and
Descending Colon

Ascending Colon

Small Intestine
and Mesentery

Pelvic Colon &

Rectum

BLADDER

See section on "PELVIS".

OTHER ORGANS

These include the gall bladder, pancreas, pelvic organs and major blood vessels. A laparotomy is indicated if there are signs of peritonitis, continuing bleeding or if the diagnosis is in doubt.

ADDITIONAL INVESTIGATIONS

X-ray of the abdomen and chest is essential in abdominal injuries. This may show gas under the diaphragm or a pleural effusion. Fractures of the transverse processes of the lumbar vertebrae are often damaged in a major abdominal injury.

Computerised tomography and ultrasound of the abdomen may show evidence of haematoma with rupture of the liver, spleen or kidney. Radioisotope scanning of the liver or other organs can also be helpful. Investigation of the urinary tract includes a cystogram which may show extravasation of urine into the extraperitoneal space as well as into the abdomen with a rupture. An intravenous pyelogram is essential for renal or retroperitoneal injuries.

Abdominal lavage, with a small catheter into the upper abdominal cavity and running in 500-1000 ml of saline, is valuable if blood, air or abdominal contents are suspected from damage to spleen, liver or gut. It is **not** helpful in retroperitoneal or bladder injuries.

It is important in all abdominal injuries to perform a laparotomy and inspect the abdominal contents if there is any doubt as to rupture or damage to any major organs.

It is also important to check the femoral pulses in severe retroperitoneal injuries, as rupture of the abdominal aorta may occur. This may sometimes mimic severe back pain and necessitate an angiogram and exploration.

ABDOMINAL INJURIES
TREATMENT

RESUSCITATION TRANSFUSION	GASTRIC TUBE PARENTERAL FLUIDS	LAPAROTOMY IF IN DOUBT

LIVER DIAPHRAGM VESSELS

SPLEEN

Diagnostic
Paracentesis

Repair or
Excise if necessary

Repair if Necessary

(S)

(S)

GALL BLADDER

Explore

KIDNEY URETER

CT Scan

PANCREAS

I.V.P.
Check
Opposite
Kidney

Explore if
Extravasation Dye

Conservative Usually

Drain (S)

(S)

OESOPHAGUS STOMACH
SMALL INTESTINE

LARGE GUT

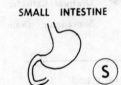

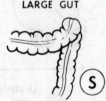

Repair / Aspiration (S)

Repair / Colostomy (S)

BLADDER INJURIES

INTRAPERITONEAL RUPTURE

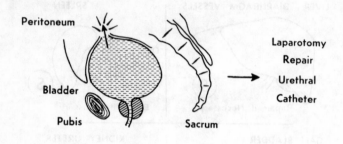

Laparotomy
Repair
Urethral
Catheter

EXTRAPERITONEAL RUPTURE

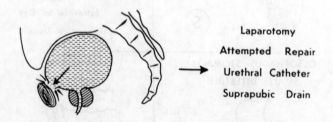

Laparotomy
Attempted Repair
Urethral Catheter
Suprapubic Drain

Urethrogram, Cystogram, and
IVP or CT Scan if Necessary
Suprapubic Catheter as well
in all Severe Bladder Injuries

URETHRAL INJURIES

MEMBRANOUS URETHRA

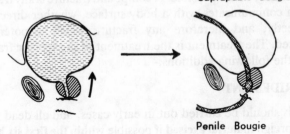

Open Bladder
Suprapubic Bougie

Penile Bougie

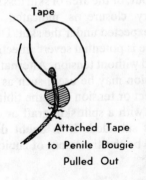

Tape

Attached Tape
to Penile Bougie
Pulled Out

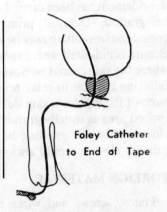

Foley Catheter
to End of Tape

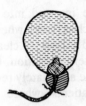

30 ml Foley Catheter

```
PENILE URETHRA
Urethrogram if Blood
     at Meatus
Pass Sterile Catheter
Repair Complete Rupture
Catheter Partial Rupture
Regular Dilatation
        Post - Operatively
```

TREATMENT OF OPEN FRACTURES

Compound fractures of large bones may lead to severe complications. These should be operated on **within** six hours of occurrence, where possible. A compound fracture is any fracture which communicates with a body surface, whether directly or indirectly, and therefore any fracture which is potentially infected. The treatment is the treatment of the specific fracture with the following additions:-

DEBRIDEMENT

This should be carried out in early cases, and all dead tissue and foreign material **excised** if possible **within the first six hours.** Primary skin closure should be attempted if adequate debridement has been carried out, or the area of skin loss should be grafted. Delayed primary closure is indicated where considerable swelling may be expected under the skin. Delayed closure is indicated where there is potential severe infection, or where the skin cannot be closed without tension. Alternatively a relieving incision to relax tension may be used, such as in the back of the calf for a skin defect or tension over the tibia. This incised area is usually grafted with a split skin graft or can be closed when the swelling has subsided. **If in doubt** delayed primary closure should **always** be the treatment of choice.

FOREIGN MATERIAL

Plates, screws and wires must **not** be inserted into open fractures **except in special cases.** These include cases where the wound is compound from within out and otherwise clean, or where vascular repair has necessitated internal fixation. Other cases are those in which fractures cannot be adequately reduced without operative fixation and in patients where early mobilisation is important.

OPEN WOUNDS AND FRACTURES

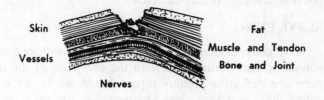

Skin

Fat

Muscle and Tendon

Vessels

Bone and Joint

Nerves

Penetration may have damaged

Brain

Chest and

Abdomen

EMERGENCY TREATMENT

PNEUMATIC SPLINT

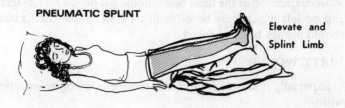

Elevate and
Splint Limb

Treat Patient
for
Shock and Haemorrhage
Respiratory Obstruction
Other Injuries

Chemotherapy
T.I.G. and Toxoid

CUT TENDONS

These, if seen, should be sutured, but it is seldom justifiable to extend the skin incision to effect a major repair in dirty wounds. Hand injuries are discussed below.

NERVE ENDS

Nerve ends, if seen, may be approximated with one or two non-absorbable sutures, but with the exception of the digital nerves, a definitive primary repair should **not** be attempted, unless there is a very clean sharp wound and micro-surgical techniques are available. The ideal time for repair in a contused or potentially infected wound is three weeks after injury, provided the wound has healed completely.

ALL but the most minor cases require admission to hospital.

FRACTURES

These should be reduced and held either by a padded back slab, or a well padded split plaster with a window cut over the wound. Excision of the dead bone should **not** be too radical lest a gap be left which may be difficult to graft. Skelecast fixation should always be considered.

DIRTY WOUNDS

Especially if muscle is involved, these may go on to infection with:-
    (a) Pyogenic Organisms, i.e., Staphylococcus
    (b) Tetanus
    (c) Gas Gangrene

GENERAL DEBRIDEMENT

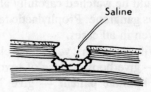

Saline

Remove All
Foreign Material
(Except Multiple
Deep Fragments
i.e. Shot Gun Pellets)

Clean Well with Saline

FAT AND MUSCLE

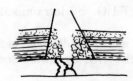

Excise All Dead Fat
and Muscle

Clean Well

Minimum Deep Sutures

LEAVE OPEN AND DELAYED PRIMARY SUTURE

TENDONS

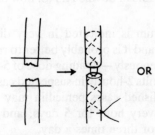

OR

Black Silk
Suture to
Anchor Tendon
and
Note Position

Suture if Easy

Secondary Suture or **Graft**
<u>Later</u> for Defects

Patients with major compound fractures should therefore be given **prophylactic** chemotherapy such as cloxacillin and ampicillin plus and **large** doses of penicillin intravenously except in suspected allergy. They should be watched carefully also, in case they develop tetanus or gas gangrene. Prophylactic tetanus toxoid or T.I.G. should be given in **all** cases.

(a) **Fully immunised patient** — if more than 2 years have elapsed since last dose of toxoid — give booster dose of toxoid.

(b) **Non-immune or partially immune patient** — give T.I.G. (Tetanus Immunoglobulin Human) **plus** a dose of adsorbed tetanus toxoid into a different site.

In addition further doses of toxoid should be given where appropriate to complete the course of immunisation.

DOSAGES OF T.I.G.

(a) **Normal Dose** — 250 I.U. of T.I.G. by intramuscular injection.

(b) **Grossly Contaminated Wound if more than 48 hours before treatment started** — 500 I.U. of T.I.G. by intramuscular injection.

(c) **Clinical Tetanus** — 4,000 I.U. of T.I.G. intravenuosly — no necessity to repeat this dosage due to half life of 3 — 4 weeks in circulation.

(d) There is **NO** indication for equine or bovine A.T.S. now that T.I.G. is available.

Occasionally gas gangrene serum is indicated in very dirty wounds, but its value is in doubt, and it is probably better to rely on huge doses of penicillin intravenously — loading dose of 5-10 million units and then 2 million units 2-hourly in suspected cases plus probenecid 0.5G. In established cases penicillin may be increased to 2-3 million units every hour for 5 days, and in addition hyperbaric oxygen two or three times a day.

GENERAL DEBRIDEMENT

BONE

Delayed Primary or Secondary Suture
in all Contaminated Wounds

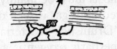

Treat Fracture
as for
Closed Injury

Excise Loose Fragments Only

Do NOT leave Large Defect

AVOID INTERNAL FIXATION

IF ALTERNATIVE MEASURES ARE AVAILABLE

USE EXTERNAL FIXATION IF INDICATED

JOINTS

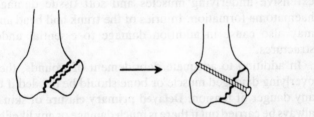

Restore Congruity

Internal Fixation if Necessary

Close Wound if Possible
with Suction Drain

It should be stressed that hyperbaric oxygen will **not** supersede adequate debridement, but it is a useful adjunct and may either save a limb or permit selective amputation at a lower level than would otherwise be possible.

In all suspected cases of gas gangrene, the wound must be **opened widely** and **left open** and all necrotic muscle excised. It must be stressed that the diagnosis must be mainly clinical and treatment should **not** be delayed until gas is seen on x-ray or a Gram stain shows the typical "Drumstick" bacteria and spores. In the case of units where hyperbaric oxygen is available, the limb may sometimes be saved, but where this is not available amputation is usually indicated to save the patient's life in proven gas gangrene, especially in the lower limb and where the patient is toxic.

PROPHYLACTIC EXPLORATION OF PUNCTURE WOUNDS

It is essential to explore and carry out adequate debridement in all puncture wounds where there is underlying muscle or bone damage. Many apparently superficial injuries of the limbs have extensive underlying muscles and soft tissue damage with haematoma formation. Injuries of the trunk and head and neck may also cause in addition damage to essential underlying structures.

In addition to adequate debridement of wounds, the fascia overlying damaged muscle or bone should be divided if there is any danger of tension. **Delayed primary closure** of skin should always be carried out if there is much damage or any likelihood of tension under the skin. Always leave a dirty contaminated wound **open** and close this later by delayed primary or secondary suture if in doubt.

SUTURING AND LACERATIONS

Full Depth

NOT Too Tight

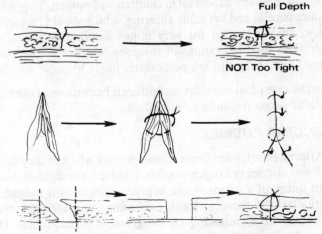

Excise Ragged Edges

Skin Graft if Necessary

METHODS OF SUTURING

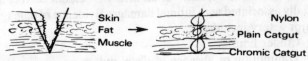

Skin — Nylon
Fat — Plain Catgut
Muscle — Chromic Catgut

Excise Skin Edges and

Devitalised Deep Tissue

DAMAGED SKIN EDGES

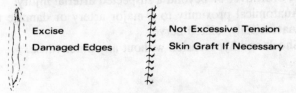

Excise
Damaged Edges

Not Excessive Tension
Skin Graft If Necessary

SUCTION DRAIN FOR ALL LARGE WOUNDS

OR DELAYED PRIMARY SUTURE

FACIAL LACERATIONS

These may gape and cause disfigurement even when small. This is particularly important in children and women. They often require careful and very fine suturing, which should be carried out in theatre except for very minor lacerations. Contused lacerations, and lacerations of the eyelids, (except when very minor) and of the lips are particularly likely to cause scarring.

In the case of **all** extensive and difficult lacerations of the face, a plastic surgeon should be consulted.

VASCULAR INJURIES

Arterial injuries are surgical emergencies whether they occur in closed injuries or in open wounds. If there is the **slightest** doubt as to injury of a major vessel, urgent exploration is indicated, particularly if there is frank ischaemia, uncontrolled open bleeding, or a pulsating or progressive haematoma. The "Doppler" ultrasound stethoscope is an invaluable aid to diagnosing blood flow and constriction in vessels.

A diagnosis of "spasm" of an artery is **seldom** correct and is usually associated with intimal damage. Evidence of damage of a major artery includes:-

(a) Colder limb.

(b) Diminution or absence of distal pulses.

(c) Increasing haematoma.

(d) Presence and/or a history of persistent arterial bleeding.

(e) A bruit over or beyond a suspected arterial injury.

(f) Anatomical proximity to a major artery or damage to an anatomically related nerve.

(g) Shock and hypotension without any other cause.

OPEN WOUNDS AND FRACTURES

SKIN COVER

SPLIT SKIN GRAFTING

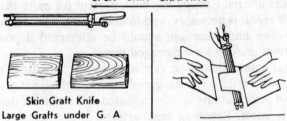

Skin Graft Knife
Large Grafts under G. A.

RELIEVING INCISION

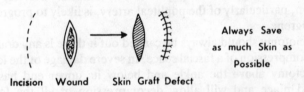

Incision   Wound   Skin Graft Defect

Always Save
as much Skin as
Possible

| V.Y. ADVANCEMENT | Z PLASTY | ROTATION FLAP |

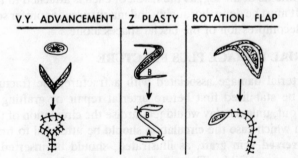

Always Cover Bone if Possible

ANGIOGRAPHY

There is a definite risk associated with angiography, and this test should **only** be used if there is doubt about the diagnosis, or where the arterial damage has been present for more than 24 hours. If repair is necessary, end to end operative suture of the artery, even under tension, should be attempted if possible rather than grafting for a damaged vessel.

Lateral suture should be carried out only for partial clean division of an artery. The danger of trauma to the intima is very real, and embolectomy is only indicated if it is certain that the intima is intact. Repair of small arteries in the vicinity of the ankle and wrist may be successful in preserving a limb which may otherwise need amputation.

It is essential to try to restore blood flow beyond the knee and elbow in damage to the popliteal and brachial arteries, as ligation, particularly of the popliteal artery, is likely to progress to gangrene.

Fasciotomy should always be carried out if there is any doubt as to compression of a fascial space. In severe damage of the leg, fibulectomy **above** the ankle and below its upper end has a limited place and will allow decompression of all the four compartments of the leg, as the fascia of each is attached to the fibula. It must be done thoroughly and many surgeons prefer soft tissue decompression of the fascial spaces alone.

ARTERIAL DAMAGE PLUS FRACTURE

In arterial damage associated with a fracture, the fracture should be stabilised first before arterial repair or grafting is carried out, unless delay would jeopardise the circulation of the limb, in which case the circulation should be attended to first.

A **reversed** vein graft, as illustrated, should be inserted if repair is not possible. There is little indication for the use of synthetic grafts in the limbs owing to the risk of infection in traumatic wounds and their lack of elasticity.

VASCULAR INJURIES

TYPES

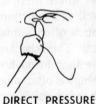

DIRECT PRESSURE BY FRACTURE

COMPRESSION UNDER FASCIA

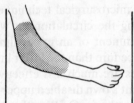

PARTIAL OR COMPLETE DIVISION

TREATMENT CLOSED INJURIES

BRACHIAL

Supracondylar Fracture

or

Severe Injury Elbow

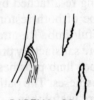

Internally Fix Explore Artery if Necessary

POPLITEAL

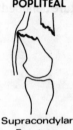

Supracondylar Fracture

or

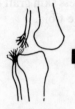

Dislocated Knee

➤ Reduce Fracture

or

Dislocation

Explore Artery

VEIN GRAFT FOR MAJOR ARTERIAL & VENOUS DAMAGE OF LIMBS

RE-ATTACHMENT OF LIMBS

In many major centres thoughout the world limbs are now being re-attached by microsurgical techniques where there is a hope of both restoring the circulation, as well as a functional useful limb. Re-attachment of an upper limb is often a much more satisfactory procedure than the lower limb. This is because upper limb prostheses are much less effective than lower limb prostheses. The patient's own disabled upper limb is often much more useful than a prosthesis. On the other hand, a good lower limb below-knee prosthesis is better than the poorly functional, badly deformed or painful existing limb of a patient. There is **therefore** much more indication for re-attachment of the upper limb, which is also more likely to regain its circulation, than in the case of the lower limb. In severe hand injuries the thumb should **always** be saved if possible where an isolated finger may not be worth saving.

It is recommended at present that the amputated limb or digit be wrapped in a sealed plastic bag. This is then put into another plastic bag containing saline and the whole package put into a container of **iced** water.

Another new method of saving limbs, which might otherwise be amputated, is by using free flap grafts. Large flaps of skin are taken from elsewhere, and anastamosed to the local blood supply by microsurgical techniques. This is particularly valuable in obtaining a full thickness skin graft over a fracture denuded of skin, paticularly over the tibia.

VASCULAR INJURIES

OPERATIVE TREATMENT

SUTURE

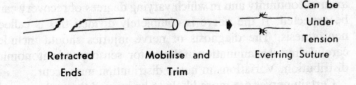

Can be
Under
Tension

| Retracted Ends | Mobilise and Trim | Everting Suture |

GRAFT

Reverse Vein

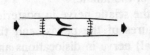

Saphenous Vein

Synthetic Graft
NOT USUALLY FOR LIMBS

MAJOR VASCULAR INJURY

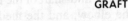

Always Explore
if Any Doubt

Colder Limb or Diminished
Distal Pulses

Increasing Haematoma or
Persisting Arterial Bleeding

Bruit Over or Beyond
Arterial Injury

Proximity Artery or Damage
Adjacent Nerve

Shock / Hypotension–No Other Cause

PERIPHERAL NERVE INJURIES

There are three grades of nerve injuries, as illustrated. Temporary physiological division only, which recovers completely, is called neurapraxia. Axonotmesis is damage of the axon in continuity and in which varying degrees of recovery can be expected. If the nerve is completely divided this is called neurotmesis. The diagnosis of nerve injuries should include careful clinical examination of the motor, sensory and autonomic distribution. Variations in nerve distribution may occur.

Certain nerves are more likely to be injured than others, and these are illustrated. In the upper limb these include the axillary (circumflex) nerve in fractures and dislocations of the shoulder, the radial nerve in fractures of the mid-shaft of the humerus, the ulnar nerve in injuries of the elbow, and the median nerve in wrist fractures and in dislocations of the lunate.

In the lower limb they include the sciatic nerve in posterior dislocations of the hip and fractures of the pelvis, and the common peroneal (lateral popliteal) nerve in dislocations and fractures of the knee and in injuries of the upper fibula.

In addition to sensory and motor examination, autonomic changes such as sweating and changes in skin texture, should be looked for, particularly in brachial plexus injuries.

Electromyographic (EMG) studies 3 weeks after injury may be valuable in assessing the likelihood of recovery of nerve injuries. In closed injuries, recovery is likely in many cases, and the speed of regeneration is approximately 1mm per day or 3cm a month. In closed injuries also, recovery can be estimated clinically by assessing the length of time taken by the nerve to reach the nearest muscle group, and adding an extra month.

PERIPHERAL NERVE INJURIES
CLASSIFICATION

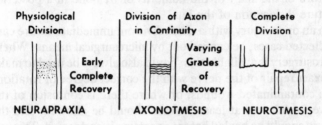

Physiological Division

Early Complete Recovery

NEURAPRAXIA

Division of Axon in Continuity

Varying Grades of Recovery

AXONOTMESIS

Complete Division

NEUROTMESIS

TREATMENT
CLOSED INJURIES

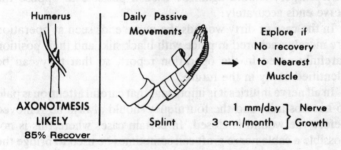

Humerus

AXONOTMESIS LIKELY 85% Recover

Daily Passive Movements

Splint

Explore if No recovery to Nearest Muscle

1 mm/day ⎤ Nerve
3 cm./month ⎦ Growth

OPEN INJURIES
Refer to Specialised Centre Early

Only Anchor Nerve Ends in Initial Wound

Slices Until Neurofibrils Seen

Suture Perineurium Without Tension

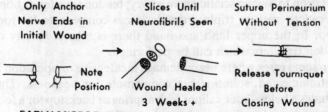

Note Position

Wound Healed 3 Weeks +

Release Tourniquet Before Closing Wound

EARLY MICROSURGERY GIVES BEST RESULTS
Immediate Primary Suture ONLY in Clean Sharp Wounds
Splint Limb to Prevent Tension

In most cases where no recovery has occurred the nerve should be explored, as it may be pressed upon by callus such as in a fracture of the shaft of the humerus or by bone in a posterior fracture dislocation of the hip.

In an open injury with a clean division, immediate suture can, in selected cases, be carried out by microsurgical means. Where microsurgery is available this should also always be used to make an exact repair of the nerve with the correct degree of rotation.

In contaminated wounds, or where there is contusion of the nerve, a delay of at least **3 weeks** should be allowed, and the wound should be healed before operation is performed. This will allow the scarring of the nerve to be completed. The nerve can then be sliced until unscarred neurofibrils are seen. Microsurgery should again be used if possible to oppose the nerve ends accurately.

In the case of dirty wounds the nerve ends seen at operation are merely anchored in place with black silk, and their position carefully noted in the operation report, so that they can be identified easily in the future.

In all nerve injuries it is important that careful attention is paid to haemostasis, and the tourniquet should always be removed before the wound is closed. In certain cases where this is not possible a cable nerve graft can sometimes be used to bridge the defect.

In cases where recovery does not take place, particularly in foot drop following sciatic nerve injury, tendon transfer or bony operations such as triple arthrodesis can compensate for foot drop. In the upper limb and hand there is a large variety of tendon transfers which can be performed.

In some cases where nerve damage is extensive or operation is contraindicated, splinting can compensate for weakness. This includes a below-knee caliper with a spring or backstop for a foot drop, or a plastic splint or other wrist or elbow supports for upper limb weakness.

PERIPHERAL NERVE INJURIES

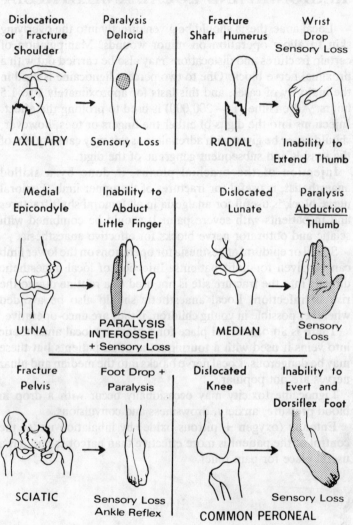

Dislocation or Fracture Shoulder → Paralysis Deltoid

AXILLARY — Sensory Loss

Fracture Shaft Humerus → Wrist Drop Sensory Loss

RADIAL — Inability to Extend Thumb

Medial Epicondyle → Inability to Abduct Little Finger

ULNA — PARALYSIS INTEROSSEI + Sensory Loss

Dislocated Lunate → Paralysis <u>Abduction</u> Thumb

MEDIAN — Sensory Loss

Fracture Pelvis → Foot Drop + Paralysis

SCIATIC — Sensory Loss Ankle Reflex

Dislocated Knee → Inability to Evert and Dorsiflex Foot

COMMON PERONEAL — Sensory Loss

See Individual Fractures For Further Details

REGIONAL AND LOCAL ANAESTHESIA

Local anaesthesia should be given directly into the overlying skin to allow operation on minor wounds. Manipulation of certain fractures and dislocations may also be carried out with a proximal nerve block. One to two percent lignocaine is used in the majority of cases, and this lasts for approximately 1 to 1.5 hours. Adrenaline (1 — 200,000) is used to prolong the effect. Injections into the digits of either the fingers or toes, however, should **never** be given with adrenaline as this may cause spasm of the vessels and subsequent gangrene of the digit.

Injection of the brachial plexus, if done by a skilled anaesthetist, is useful for fractures of the upper limb. Femoral nerve block is useful for analgesia in all femoral shaft fractures and in patients with severe pain. It should be combined with sciatic and obturator nerve blocks for effective anaesthesia.

Spinal or epidural anaesthesia for operations on the lower limb can be given for unfit patients. Injection of local anaesthetic directly into the fracture site is not used as a routine due to the risk of infection. Local anaesthetic should also be avoided wherever possible in young children, if they are unco-operative.

There is an occasional place for a block by local anaesthetic into veins if used with a tourniquet in adult patients but these may be dangerous. Local nerve blocks into the median and ulnar nerves are not popular.

Lignocaine toxicity may occasionally occur with a drop in blood pressure, anxiety, drowsiness and convulsions.

Entonox (oxygen + nitrous oxide) by inhalation under the control of the patient is more effective than narcotics and has a useful place for pain relief.

REGIONAL AND LOCAL ANAESTHESIA

LOCAL WOUNDS

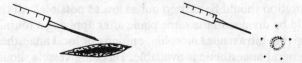

BRACHIAL PLEXUS | DIGITAL NERVES

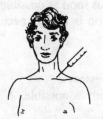

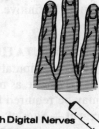

**NEVER Adrenaline   With Digital Nerves
USE 1-2% XYLOCAINE**

LOWER LIMB

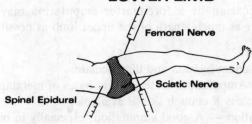

Femoral Nerve

Sciatic Nerve

Spinal Epidural

**NOTE - AVOID LOCAL ANAESTHESIA IN
UNCOOPERATIVE CHILDREN**

AMPUTATIONS

EMERGENCY AMPUTATIONS

In trapped limbs which cannot be freed at accident sites, amputation should be carried out as low as possible. All tissues should be divided in the same plane after applying a tourniquet and giving **intravenous** morphia, entonox or local anaesthesia if no general anaesthetic is available. Bleeding vessels should be tied off if possible or the tourniquet should be let off for 5 minutes each hour provided an intravenous drip is in situ and the pulse and blood pressure are stable. The limb should be elevated and a local pressure bandage applied as soon as possible instead of a tourniquet. Definitive amputation is always necessary in hospital.

UPPER LIMB AMPUTATIONS

Fingers — Radical amputation if necessary.

Thumb — Always save as much thumb as possible. A bone or skin graft may be required later.

Arm & Forearm — Sites of election for optimum limb fitting are 2/3rds the distance down the humerus and 2/3rds the distance below the olecranon.

Shoulder — Save head and neck of humerus if possible or at least acromion. Occasionally a forequarter amputation may be necessary. **Save** as much length of the upper limb as possible.

LOWER LIMB

Toes — Use racquet incision and disarticulate.

Metatarsals — Amputations at necks or at bases of metatarsals may be satisfactory if enough skin is available.

Symes Amputation — A good amputation, especially in older patients. It is, however, cosmetically unacceptable to most women.

Below Knee — Ideally 12cm below tibial plateau but even 6 cm or less is acceptable. Bevel tibia anteriorly and cut fibula 2 cm shorter than tibia and bevel laterally.

EMERGENCY AMPUTATIONS

INSTRUMENTS

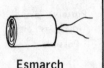

Scalpel
Artery Forceps
Sutures and
Needles
Dressings and
Bandages

Esmarch
Tourniquet or
Pneumatic Tourniquet

Miniature 15 cm. Hacksaw

LIMB TRAPPED AT ACCIDENT SITE

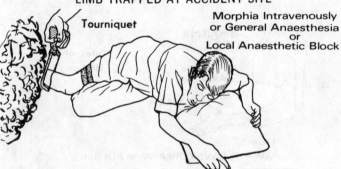

Tourniquet

Morphia Intravenously
or General Anaesthesia
or
Local Anaesthetic Block

Divide All Tissues as low as Possible
Do not attempt Flaps

Dressing
+
Crepe
Bandage

Release Tourniquet
At Least Every
One Hour

Leave Off Completely
if Possible

Tie Off Major
Vessels if Time
Allows

Leave Wound Open
and Pressure Bandage

Direct Pressure
+ Elevation

ALWAYS REQUIRES DEFINITIVE AMPUTATION IN HOSPITAL

AMPUTATIONS

UPPER LIMB

Preserve Joint if Possible

Radical if Necessary

Strength— Men
Cosmesis—Women

Preserve as Much as Possible

FINGERS

THUMB

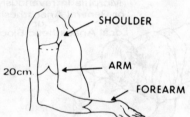

SHOULDER

ARM

FOREARM

20cm

17cm.

Sites of Election

ALWAYS SAVE FOREARM IF POSSIBLE

LOWER LIMB

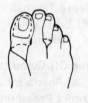

TOES

NECK METATARSALS

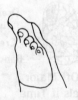

BASES METATARSALS

AMPUTATIONS
LOWER LIMB

SYME'S

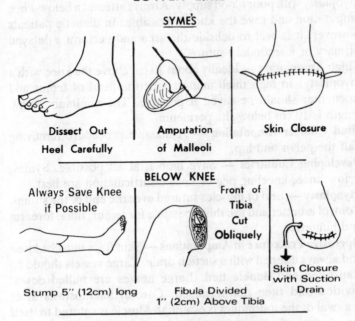

Dissect Out
Heel Carefully

Amputation
of Malleoli

Skin Closure

BELOW KNEE

Always Save Knee
if Possible

Front of
Tibia
Cut
Obliquely

Skin Closure
with Suction
Drain

Stump 5" (12cm) long

Fibula Divided
1" (2cm) Above Tibia

THROUGH AND ABOVE KNEE

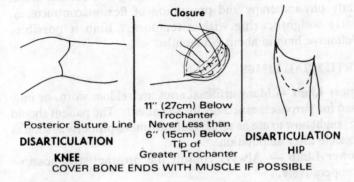

Posterior Suture Line

**DISARTICULATION
KNEE**

Closure

11" (27cm) Below
Trochanter
Never Less than
6" (15cm) Below
Tip of
Greater Trochanter

**DISARTICULATION
HIP**

COVER BONE ENDS WITH MUSCLE IF POSSIBLE

Use anterior 2/3rds posterior 1/3rd flaps for simple artificial limbs. A large posterior flap may sometimes be indicated in a myoplasty with poor blood supply. Always attempt a below-knee amputation and save the knee if possible. In diabetic patients however, it is best to debride the area and perform a delayed primary or a secondary suture.

Thigh Amputation — Ideally about 10 cm above the knee with a myoplasty. In high thigh amputations the head of femur and trochanter should be saved if possible. The minimum stump length is 10 cm below the perineum.

Hind Quarter Amputation — A massive procedure removing half the pelvis and hip.

Developing Countries — Save limb if at all possible. Symes, below knee, kneeling peg or knee disarticulation are best.

Myoplasty — End of muscles sutured **over** the end of the stump. Control is better and use this if possible for femur, tibia, forearm and humerus.

Operative Procedure in Amputations — Skin flaps must be loose and **always** drained with a suction drain. Large vessels should be transfixed and **double** tied. Large nerves are pulled down, divided and then diathermised. Careful haemostasis after removal of the tourniquet is essential. Muscle is sutured to itself over bone ends after trimming. Always use a suction drain.

Post-Operative Care — Careful bandaging and suction drain. Early physiotherapy and prevention of flexion contractures. Early weightbearing with a temporary limb if possible. Definitive limb in about 2-3 months.

ARTIFICIAL LIMBS

Upper Limb — Many artificial arms are seldom worn, or only used for purposes, especially in old patients. The patient should be taught how to use an upper limb prosthesis properly as soon as possible after amputation.

Lower Limb — Always consult the prosthetist if possible preoperatively.

AMPUTATIONS
DEVELOPING COUNTRIES

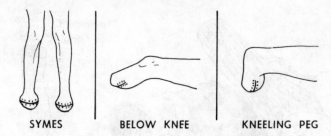

SYMES   BELOW KNEE   KNEELING PEG

SAVE AS MUCH ARM AS POSSIBLE

DRAIN WELL OR SECONDARY SUTURE

MYOPLASTY

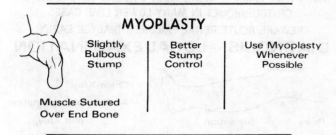

Slightly Bulbous Stump

Better Stump Control

Use Myoplasty Whenever Possible

Muscle Sutured Over End Bone

POST OPERATIVE CARE

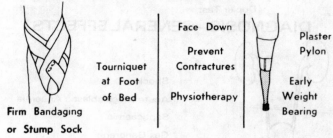

Firm Bandaging or Stump Sock

Tourniquet at Foot of Bed

Face Down

Prevent Contractures

Physiotherapy

Plaster Pylon

Early Weight Bearing

ALWAYS DP N WITH SUCTION DRAIN

CRUSH SYNDROME
CAUSATION

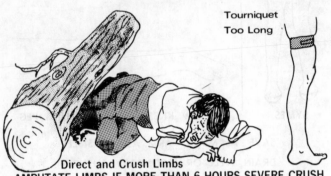

Tourniquet
Too Long

Direct and Crush Limbs

**AMPUTATE LIMBS IF MORE THAN 6 HOURS SEVERE CRUSH
OR TOURNIQUET IN MANY LOWER LIMB CASES
BEWARE ACUTE RENAL FAILURE - DIALYSE EARLY**

DIAGNOSIS -- LOCAL EXAMINATION

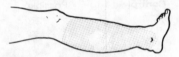

Pallor	Sensation	Chest Xray
Power	Tenseness	Abdominal Examination and Xray
Pulses	Fascial Compartments	Full Blood Investigation
	Dopler Test	Including Coombes Test

DIAGNOSIS - GENERAL EFFECTS

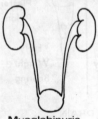

Myoglobinuria
Renal Failure

Shock
Acute Megaloblastic Anaemia
Septicaemia
Gas Gangrene
Pyogenic Infection

CRUSH SYNDROME
TREATMENT
PROPHYLAXIS

LOCAL   GENERAL

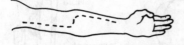

Split Tight Fascial Sheaths Early

Avoid Prolonged Tourniquets

Blood Transfusion
S.P.P.S.   Early to
Sodium Bicarbonate   Victim
Oxygen

MAINTAIN URINE OUTPUT   RENAL DIALYSIS EARLY

TREATMENT
FASCIOTOMY

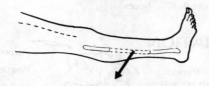

Split Flexor Sheath   Remove Mid 1/3 Fibula

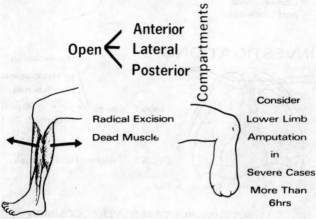

Open ← Anterior
       Lateral   Compartments
       Posterior

Radical Excision
Dead Muscle

Consider
Lower Limb
Amputation
in
Severe Cases
More Than
6hrs

POST TRAUMATIC SYNDROME
FAT EMBOLUS

HISTORY

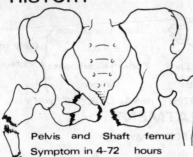

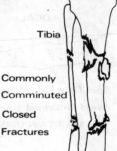

Tibia

Commonly
Comminuted
Closed
Fractures

Pelvis and Shaft femur
Symptom in 4-72 hours

EXAMINATION

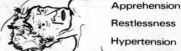

Tachypnoea Pyrexia
Petechial Rash sometimes
— Anterior Axillary Fold
— Conjunctivae
— and Elsewhere

Apprehension
Restlessness
Hypertension

INVESTIGATIONS

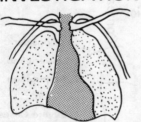

Hypercapnia
or Hypocapnia
Hypoxaemia

Blood Gases $PO_2 < 65$mm Hg
Breathing Air

ECG - Right Heart Strain

'Snow Storm' Chest x-ray

SUBCLINICAL CASES VERY COMMON

POST TRAUMATIC SYNDROME
PROPHYLAXIS

Avoid Hypovolaemia

Replace Blood Loss

High Oxygenation

Drip Bottle

Splint Injured Limbs Early

Minimal Reaming of Long Bones

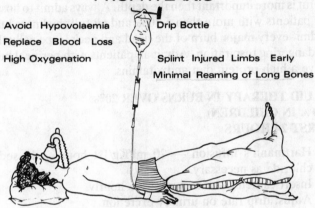

TREATMENT

HIGH OXYGENATION
Intubate or Intranasal Oxygen
or Efficient Mask for Constant
Positive Airways Pressure

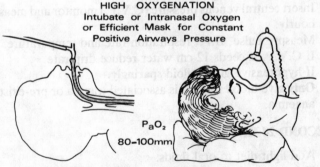

P_aO_2
80–100mm

Correct Anaemia – Packed Cells
Steroids – Dexamethasone
Very Large Doses I.V. Slowly
? Heparin – ? Trasylol

MONITOR PATIENT WITH BLOOD GASES
AND CHEST XRAY

BURNS

Careful assessment and observation is essential. The area burnt is more important then the depth. Always admit to hospital all patients with more than 5-10% and **all** full thickness burns. Admit every **major** burn of the head and neck, especially those endangering respiration. Admit all patients with perineal burns. Give a high protein diet and vitamins.

FLUID THERAPY IN BURNS OVER 20% (10% IN CHILDREN)
FIRST 24 HOURS

1. Hartmann's infusion — 20 ml/Kg/1st hour. Add sodium chloride as necessary.
2. Insert catheter — measure urine hourly.
3. Adjust drip rate on urinary excretion.
   (a) Less 0.5 ml/Kg/hr — increase rate.
   (b) More 1 ml/Kg/hr — decrease rate.
4. Insert central venous pressure (C.V.P.) monitor and measure hourly.
5. Measure pulse, B.P., respiration rate and temperature.
6. If C.V.P. exceeds 12 cm water reduce drip rate.
7. If hypotensive give colloid **sparingly.**
8. **Only** give blood if there is associated trauma or pre-existent anaemia.

SECOND 24 HOURS

1. Add light diet to oral fluids.
2. Concentrated albumin, electrolyte solution and 5% glucose according to the serum electrolytes.

AFTER 48 HOURS

1. Increase oral intake of high calorie diet.
2. Start hyperalimentation regime should oral intake be insufficient.
3. Potassium chloride and amino acid infusions if required.

ASSESSMENT IN BURNS

RULE OF 3

(Applied to Rule of 9)

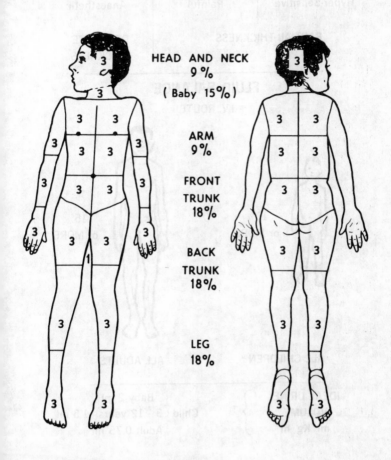

HEAD AND NECK
9 %

(Baby 15%)

ARM
9%

FRONT
TRUNK
18%

BACK
TRUNK
18%

LEG
18%

BURNS

DEPTH OF BURN

Bright Red Dry Hyper-Sensitive	Mottled Red Moist Painful	White or Black Dry Anaesthetic
PARTIAL THICKNESS		**COMPLETE THICKNESS**

FLUID BALANCE

I.V. ROUTE

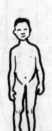

10%
or MORE

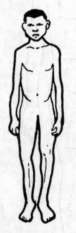

15%
or MORE

ALL CHILDREN   **ALL ADULTS**

IDEAL URINE VOLUME ml/Kg/hr	Baby 2 ml Child (3 - 12 years) 1.5 ml Adult 0.75 ml

BURNS

OPEN TREATMENT

MOST BURNS

No Dressings
I.V. Fluids

Netting
Cradles
Rest Burnt
Area

APPLICATION

Silver Sulphadiazine

Insecticide

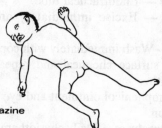

Prevent Anaemia
Check Hb every 3rd Day

LOCAL MANAGEMENT

Sterile Theatre
Clean with Cetavlon
Aspirate Blisters
Prevent Infection

Graft

When Slough Separates or
Remove Slough by 21st day
Homograft from Relative
Temporary Dressing in
Large Burns

CLOSED TREATMENT

Wrap
Each
Finger

Pressure
Over
Gauze

Hands

Minor Burns
Infected Wounds
Eye Lids
Circumferential Burns
Separated Eschar

SPECIAL BURNS AND COMPLICATIONS

Burns of Hands — Elevate and dress with silver sulphadiazine cream with hand in plastic bag or disposable plastic glove with wrist extended, M.P. joints flexed and I.P. joints extended. Daily physiotherapy. Early excision and grafting if necessary.

Respiratory Burns — Endotracheal tube.

Electrical Burns — Excise immediately and graft in full thickness.

Chemical Burns — Wash immediately with copious amounts of water to remove surface chemical and repeat frequently by showering or a bath.

Cornea — Chloramphenicol ointment and eye pad and consult ophthalmic surgeon.

Prevention of Contractures — Daily physiotherapy, splinting and early grafting.

Circumferential Burns — These may cause peripheral circulatory embarrassment due to oedema beneath inelastic eschar. Careful observation and escharotomy and/or fasciotomy if paraesthesia, absence of pulse, pain or colour change or other evidence of compression.

Flexor Area — e.g., neck, axilla, elbow and knee. Early splint and skin graft to prevent contracture. Replace by full thickness or thick split skin 3-6 months after burn.

Infection & Toxaemia — Treat anaemia with blood (check Hb. 2 x/wk) plus chemotherapy and frequent change of dressings. Early excision and grafting. Check bacterial flora. Skin graft will not take in presence of haemolytic streptococci. Silver sulphadiazine for infection.

Venous Thrombosis & Embolism — Early movements and ambulation essential, especially with lower limbs.

Cosmesis — Early reconstruction and grafting, especially face.

Note: Never underestimate the severity of a burn.

Patients may die with a 20% burn if not properly treated.

BURNS

COMPLICATIONS

Tracheostomy
or Intubation

RESPIRATORY OBSTRUCTION

Flex Joints and Elevate
FROZEN HANDS

Daily Physiotherapy

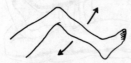

Splinting
Grafting
CONTRACTURES

Treat Anaemia
Chemotherapy
Dressings
Early Grafting

**INFECTION AND
TOXAEMIA**

Early
Movements
and
Ambulation

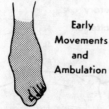

**VENOUS THROMBOSIS
AND EMBOLISM**

Early Grafting
Later Reconstruction
DEFORMITY

RADIATION INJURIES
ATOMIC BOMB   NUCLEAR REACTOR

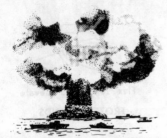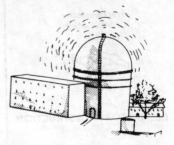

DIRECT INJURIES

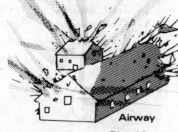

Airway   Splint   Pressure Bandage

Blood Loss   Treat Shock   for Bleeding

BLAST INJURIES

Corneal Damage   Respiratory

Ear Drum   Resuscitation

Lungs

Frothy Blood

TREAT SHOCK

I.V. DRIP

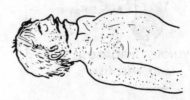

RADIATION INJURIES
BURNS

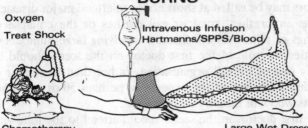

Oxygen

Treat Shock

Intravenous Infusion
Hartmanns/SPPS/Blood

Chemotherapy
Space Blanket
Silver Sulphadiazine   Locally

Large Wet Dressings
for Large Areas
with Pain

RADIATION CONTAMINATION

Shave
Contaminated
Hair

Shower
Without
Clothing

Scrub
Thoroughly

Use
Radiation
Monitor
if Available

<u>WATCH FOR LATE EFFECTS</u>

1—4 Weeks Later

Immediate
Effects

Immediate Effects	1—4 Weeks Later
Nausea	Desquamation
Vomiting	CNS Toxicity
Diarrhoea	Aplastic Anaemia
Toxaemia	Renal Failure
Low WBC	Alopecia
Haemorrhage	Pyrexia
Sterility	

Dispose of all clothing and effects

Plastic Bag or Metal Trunk

WEAR GLOVES   ISOLATE FROM

OTHER PATIENTS

If Material Ingested Collect Excreta
and Vomiting and Store for Disposal

Wash Open Wounds

WATCH FOR LATE RADIATION FALLOUT

MANAGEMENT OF MASS DISASTERS

Doctors may be called at short notice to attend major disasters such as air crashes, road or rail crashes or the collapse of buildings or mines. In all disasters involving large numbers of casualties the role of the first doctor on the scene should be initially one of overall **organisation,** rather than treatment of individual casualties at the expense of perhaps 50 or 100 other patients who will thereby be neglected.

The first doctor on the scene should attend to the following priorities until relieved by a more senior colleague or by additional help:-

ORGANISATION AND COMMUNICATION

(a) Have **police, ambulance, fire brigade** (including crash vans) and extra **doctors** and **nurses** been summoned and **hospitals notified?**

(b) Has **traffic** been diverted to save subsequent crashes?

(c) Has an **emergency first aid post** been set up in a **central** position away from danger of explosions? Has this post, and the doctor taking charge, a police officer with him with a **two-way transmitter** to ensure communication at **all** times?

(d) Have all available personnel at the crash site been organised to call for additional help, to administer first aid systematically, and look for survivors?

FIRST AID TO THE SEVERELY INJURED

The doctor in charge, if the **only** doctor available, should normally **remain** at his temporary first aid post, and casualties, suitably splinted where necessary, should be brought to him for resuscitation and treatment.

If there is more than one doctor available, the most senior should remain at the first aid and communication post with as much help as needed, while the more junior (accompanied by a police officer with a two-way radio, and by as many helpers as possible) should rapidly examine the injured at the scene of the crash, but should **leave** actual splinting or first aid treatment to those accompanying him until he has seen all the severe cases. Those patients in need of **immediate** life-saving measures should be treated first, and transported as soon as possible to the first aid post.

MANAGEMENT OF MINOR INJURIES

These patients should be transported or sent back to the central clearing station for first aid dressing and splints prior to transport to hospital.

TYPE OF FIRST AID

In mass disasters the accent should be on speed and resuscitation, with priorities in the life-saving measures of clearing airways, and maintaining respiratory and cardiac functions, stopping haemorrhage, the treatment of shock and the splinting of limbs by pneumatic splints where possible. Support of neck or spine where fractures or dislocations are suspected is important **before** moving. Wounds and burns should be covered by large clean "shell" dressings, or, failing this, by any large clean piece of cloth. **No** attempt should be made to clean or suture wounds or apply special dressings except in special circumstances.

LABELLING OF PATIENTS AND ADMINISTRATION OF DRUGS

All patients treated should be labelled, and different coloured labels will usually be provided in disasters depending on whether the patient is an emergency, a routine injury or dead.

It is essential that all those requiring drugs have the dose and time noted and that drugs should be given **intravenously** where possible.

In the case of mass casualties only a red (life threatening), green (other casualty), white with black stripe (dead), label should be attached but not written on, and details completed in the Casualty Clearing Station.

NOTIFICATION OF HOSPITALS AND TRANSPORT OF PATIENTS

In mass disasters involving large numbers of patients the careful distribution of patients to hospitals best able to deal with them should be planned where feasible. It is obviously ridiculous to rush patients to the nearest hospital when this may not have the facilities, staff or beds to cope with them. The use of helicopters where available and the transport of patients with head injuries, for instance, to centres with neurosurgeons, and those with severe chest injuries to a hospital where thoracic surgical procedures can be carried out, will obviously be in the best interests of all.

The doctor in charge must decide not only on priorities of transport of patients, but make sure that the patient is fit to travel. He should also inform the hospitals as soon as possible so that the appropriate specialists can be notified and **theatres, resuscitation facilities** and **beds** prepared. It is also essential that supportive facilities such as **blood bank, radiology** and **pathology** facilities, both at hospital and at city or national level, be put on full alert until the extent of the disaster is known.

COMMUNICATIONS

It is essential that radio stations announcing such disasters give telephone numbers for information of relatives, quite **distinct** from those of hospital switchboards, as switchboards will be rapidly jammed to the detriment of the emergency services.

The provision of radio links between police and ambulance **direct** to hospitals would do much to improve communications, and this should be planned. It is also essential that individual hospitals should designate a senior doctor to take charge of the reception and organisation of casualties, their assessment and their subsequent disposal. Each hospital must also have both an internal and external disaster plan.

RECEPTION OF CASUALTIES AT HOSPITAL

At individual hospitals the reception and treatment of casualties often requires considerable improvement. Each Accident and Emergency Centre requires, for instance, action cards for each member of staff summarising on **one** card his or her role in a major disaster. There should, in addition, be someone with both clinical and administrative experience in overall charge of organising the reception and distribution of casualties and the organisation of staff. This person, who should be called the Director of Accident & Emergency Services, should **not** usually either examine or treat individual emergencies. This should be left to a triage officer (surgeon or anaesthetist) and those responsible for resuscitation such as an experienced anaesthetist. The management of a disaster should, wherever possible, be left to senior clinical staff such as anaesthetists and surgeons, and adequate staff must always be put on alert or called in early. Specialists in all the major disciplines should make themselves immediately available, in case of need.

SOFT TISSUE INJURIES

Soft tissue injuries are extremely common, particularly following athletic injuries. The disabilities from some relatively minor soft tissue injuries, however, can be quite severe, and are often treated badly and late. A vicious circle of pathology is set up, often with the formation of a haematoma followed by lack of use which in turn leads to rapid muscle wasting. This causes ligamentous instability which if not treated early may go on to further trauma, joint effusion and sometimes joint stiffness.

All haematomas, if small, should be treated with wool and crepe bandage, ice, support and elevation. If large, they often need evacuation and drainage. Certain newer drugs may help with the dispersal of a haematoma. Early active exercises to help to disperse both haematoma and oedema fluid plus support, are essential.

Minor muscular tears and ligamentous sprains may require ice, a crepe bandage and wool followed by exercises. Minor strains and sprains may also require some support initially.

Occasionally, after soft tissue injuries associated with a fracture or dislocation, myositis ossificans or traumatic ossification may occur, particularly if there is any degree of paralysis of the limb. This is best treated with **rest** rather than exercises **until** the new bone growth has become quiescent. It may then occasionally require excision.

In chronic strain or sprains, injection of a local anaesthetic, plus hydrocortisone acetate, may be indicated into the tender area. There are dangers of tendon and ligament rupture. Intra-articular steroids into the knee or hip must **never** be given except in special cases due to the risk of an arthropathy.

SOFT TISSUE INJURIES

HAEMATOMA

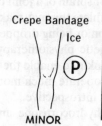

Crepe Bandage
Ice

(P)

MINOR

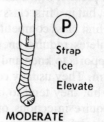

(P)

Strap
Ice
Elevate

MODERATE

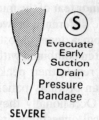

(S)

Evacuate
Early
Suction
Drain
Pressure
Bandage

SEVERE

MUSCULAR TEARS

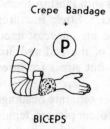

Crepe Bandage
+

(P)

BICEPS

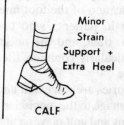

Minor
Strain
Support +
Extra Heel

CALF

Radiant Heat
Exercises
Muscular
Re-education
and
Stretches

BACK

OTHER INJURIES

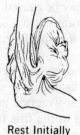

Rest Initially
**TRAUMATIC
OSSIFICATION**

Tender
Swelling

Radial
Styloid

(S)

Hydrocortisone and
Local Anaesthetics
if Necessary.
**DE QUERVAIN'S
TENOVAGINITIS**

Tendons Fingers

Extensor Mechanism

Knee

Tendo Achillis

**SEE RELEVANT
SECTIONS**

MINOR ATHLETIC INJURIES

The athlete may only present with a minor sprain of a joint or minor tear of the muscle, but in a first class athlete this may make the difference between first class competition or being dropped from a team. Most athletes require energetic physiotherapy, often combined with supports to knee and ankle to enable them to regain their peak form. They usually co-operate much more than ordinary patients, but they tend to be introspective.

Occasionally they require injections of hydrocortisone and local anaesthetic into a tender area which is not resolving by other means. Care must be taken, however, that this is **only** into a muscle or ligament and not into the joint itself.

Pain under the foot may require supports with Plastazote and with intrinsic re-education of the foot muscles. Stress fractures are not uncommon in patients who take up unaccustomed exercise. The fibula, tibia, and the necks of the 2nd and 3rd metatarsals are particularly common sites but stress fractures may occur elsewhere.

Many of these injuries are discussed under separate headings and these include damage to the menisci in soccer players, tennis or golf elbow in tennis and golf players, and tendinitis or rupture of the tendo calcaneus in athletes.

Back strain is particularly common in the lower lumbar spine. Shoulder "capsulitis" and "frozen shoulder" may be caused by C5/6 pressure in cervical spondylosis. Examination and treatment of the **cervical spine,** as well as **the shoulder,** is essential.

Most injuries merely require ice, support, exercises, heat, massage and a skin counter irritant. In acute ligamentous and muscular injuries and even some fractures, ice wrapped in a plastic bag and a towel may diminish swelling in the first few hours of injury. In convalescence, active and passive exercises and stretching, plus support if necessary, are essential before returning to sport.

MINOR ATHLETIC INJURIES

LEG

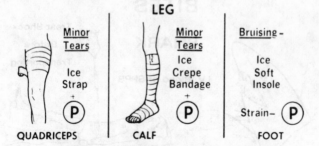

<u>Minor Tears</u>	<u>Minor Tears</u>	Bruising –
Ice Strap + (P)	Ice Crepe Bandage + (P)	Ice Soft Insole
		Strain – (P)
QUADRICEPS	CALF	FOOT

SEE KNEE AND ANKLE FOR MAJOR INJURIES

ARM

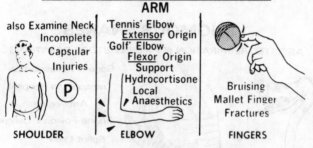

also Examine Neck Incomplete Capsular Injuries (P)	'Tennis' Elbow <u>Extensor</u> Origin 'Golf' Elbow <u>Flexor</u> Origin Support Hydrocortisone Local Anaesthetics	Bruising Mallet Finger Fractures
SHOULDER	ELBOW	FINGERS

SEE UPPER LIMB FOR MAJOR INJURIES

BACK

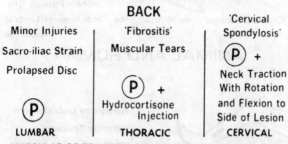

Minor Injuries Sacro-iliac Strain Prolapsed Disc (P)	'Fibrositis' Muscular Tears (P) + Hydrocortisone Injection	'Cervical Spondylosis' (P) + Neck Traction With Rotation and Flexion to Side of Lesion
LUMBAR	THORACIC	CERVICAL

MUSCULAR RE-EDUCATION TO PREVENT RECURRENCES
TEMPORARILY BACK OR CERVICAL SUPPORT IF NECESSARY

FIRST AID
BITES

SHARK

I.V. Blood or SPPS

Treat Shock
Before
Transporting

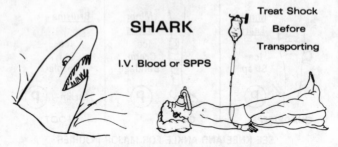

Direct Pressure or Tourniquet to Stop Bleeding

VENOMOUS SNAKES

ASSISTED RESPIRATION IF PATIENT STOPS BREATHING

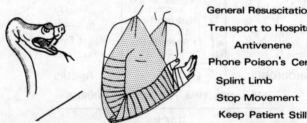

General Resuscitation
Transport to Hospital
Antivenene
Phone Poison's Centre
Splint Limb
Stop Movement
Keep Patient Still
Ice Pack around Limb if
Available

Firm Crepe Bandage over Whole Limb

ANIMAL AND HUMAN

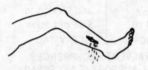

Adequate Debridement
Tetanus Toxoid ±
T.I.G.
Antibiotics

Rabies Vaccine if Indicated

FIRST AID
STINGS

JELLY FISH

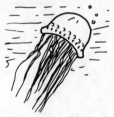

Vinegar or Weak Acid

SPIDER

Treat as for Snake Bite

BEE

Remove Sting Sideways

Alkali Locally

Aspirin

WASP

Vinegar or Weak Acid

Locally

GENERAL TREATMENT

SHOCK

Clear Airway   I.V. Fluids if Necessary

Oxygen

ANAPHYLAXIS

Adrenaline

Antihistamines

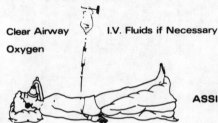

**ASSISTED VENTILATION
IF NECESSARY**

GENERAL PRINCIPLES

INTRODUCTION TO FRACTURES AND DISLOCATIONS

Fractures may occur in normal or abnormal bone and in the adult or the child. They can be caused by a variety of different forces. Each of these can cause its own pattern of fractures or dislocations, and its own complications. The overlying skin and soft tissue including blood vessels, nerves, muscles, tendons and ligaments may also be damaged and the complications of these must be looked for, not only at the site of the fracture but also distal to this.

The whole patient must be examined in any injury, as there may be signs of blood loss and pain leading to shock. Other injuries which may occur include the brain, facial skeleton, eyes, spinal cord, nerves, lung, heart, major vessels and the contents of the abdominal cavity. The late effects of trauma include toxaemia, fat embolus, gangrene, as well as infection, and the crush syndrome. These are all illustrated.

Causation of Fracture — Transverse and oblique forces may respectively lead to transverse and oblique fractures and these, in turn, are reduced by the opposite force. Crush fractures are usually caused by direct trauma. Children's bones have a different pattern of management and complications which have been described. Old people are particularly prone to Colles fracture and fractures of the neck of the humerus and hip. Patients with pathological bone, particularly with secondary deposits from carcinoma in the femur, humerus and spine, may fracture with minimal force.

Healing of Fractures — The healing of fractures is influenced by many factors, and these include the blood supply of the bone, movement, soft tissue interposition between fracture ends, age and nutrition of the patient, overlying soft tissue and skin damage, and infection.

Examination of Patients — This should include not only the **site** of the fracture with particular consideration of the skin, overlying soft tissue and the bone and joint itself, but also the limb **distal** to the fracture. This is in particular regard to vascular, neurological and bony damage. The **whole patient** must also be carefully assessed for other injuries and for complications.

Management of Injuries — The principles of management are described throughout this book. The important aspects of management can be divided into the management of the **whole patient** and the treatment of the **fracture itself,** together with any **complications.**

It can also be divided into **first aid** and **resuscitation, definitive treatment** and **rehabilitation.**

A simple guide to healing times of fractures is illustrated. Most **major fractures of major** bones take about 3 months to unite in adults. Children unite much faster than adults, and oblique fractures unite faster than transverse ones. The majority of fractures of small bones, with notable exceptions such as the scaphoid, unite in 3 weeks, as do bones with a good blood supply such as the clavicle, neck of humerus and ribs.

Modern treatment with lightweight waterproof skelecasts, instead of plaster, will speed up fracture healing. Internal fixation of many fractures will permit more movement, better reduction and earlier mobility. These include fractures of the hip, the femur, tibia and radius and ulna, as well as the ankle and elbow. Pathological fractures treated with internal fixation and cement will also allow early mobility. The main risk of internal fixation is infection, and internal fixation should be avoided in compound fractures except in special cases.

INJURIES ON THE ROAD

Emergency management of vehicle accidents, together with a list of the emergency equipment, is listed at the end of this book.

One of the first actions of those arriving at the scene of an accident is to make sure that oncoming traffic from both sides is suitably warned. Too many patients and rescuers have been injured or killed by oncoming traffic by omitting this precaution. If necessary, victims should be moved to a safe place by the side of the road out of danger from oncoming traffic.

It is important that the likely injuries which may be sustained by the driver, passengers, pedestrians and others should be looked for specifically and treated. Efforts should also be made to resuscitate and splint patients before taking them to hospital.

All unconscious patients should be placed on the side and given a simple neck support, if available. If this is not available a towel around the neck, lightly applied, will act as an emergency splint. The driver or passengers trapped in a car with likely spinal injury should be strapped onto a simple, short spinal board, or failing this, lifted carefully with back straight or hyper-extended but **never** flexed.

Fractures of the upper limb are best treated with a simple triangular sling. Fractures of the hip, femur or tibia should be treated with the injured leg tied to the uninjured leg with three triangular slings made into bandages as illustrated under "Emergency Splinting".

All cigarettes should be extinguished before a crashed vehicle is approached. It is important also to look for any victims who may have been thrown to one side of the road into the undergrowth.

125

INJURIES ON THE ROAD
CAR ACCIDENTS

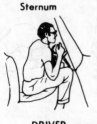

Sternum

DRIVER

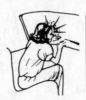

Head Injuries

DRIVER AND PASSENGER

Fracture Patella
Posterior Dislocation Hip

ALL OCCUPANTS

Crush
Fracture
Thoracic Spine

Whiplash
Cervical Spine

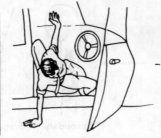

Multiple
Injuries
–Thrown out
of Car

OTHER ACCIDENTS

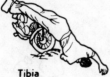

Brachial Plexus

Tibia

MOTOR CYCLE

Multiple Injuries

BICYCLE

Fracture Tibia
Other Injuries

PEDESTRIAN

TYPES OF FRACTURE
DIRECT TRAUMA

| Bumper | Comminuted | Fall on Calcaneus | Crush |

AVOID EARLY WEIGHT BEARING

PATHOLOGICAL BONE

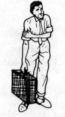 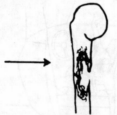 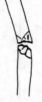

Minimal Force → Secondary Deposit   Fragilitas Ossium   Senile Osteoporosis

EARLY MOBILISATION

CHILDREN

Poor History 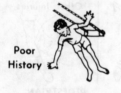 →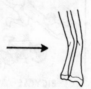

X-ray Both Sides   Greenstick   Slipped Epiphysis

EARLY REDUCTION

TYPES OF FRACTURE
DIRECT OR INDIRECT TRAUMA

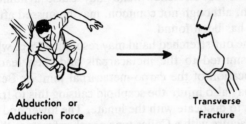

Abduction or
Adduction Force

Transverse
Fracture

REDUCE BY ADDUCTION OR ABDUCTION

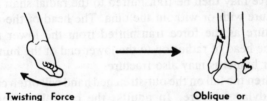

Twisting Force

Oblique or
Spiral Fracture

REDUCE BY TWISTING

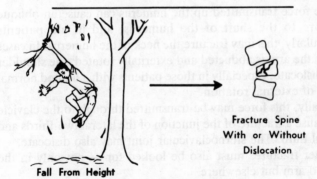

Fall From Height

Fracture Spine
With or Without
Dislocation

TREAT COMPLICATIONS

FALLS ON THE OUTSTRETCHED HAND

Falls on the out-stretched hand may cause a number of injuries which, although not common, may be missed after the first fracture has been found.

A fall on the out-stretched hand may result in a force which is initially transmitted to the metacarpals and then lead to a fracture dislocation of the carpo-metacarpal joint or Bennetts fracture. It may also injure the scaphoid causing this to fracture or half of this to dislocate with the lunate. The lower end of the radius may fracture with a Colles type or other fracture through the wrist.

The force may then be transmitted to the radial shaft which may fracture with or without the ulna. The head of the radius may fracture as the force transmitted from the lower radius crushes the head of radius on to the lower end of the humerus. The lower humerus may also fracture.

In children the fall on the out-stretched hand will often cause a supracondylar fracture. In adults, the capitellum may be fractured or the whole lower end of the humerus may be shattered.

The force transmitted up the humerus can cause an oblique fracture to the shaft of the humerus, and in old patients particularly, this may fracture the neck of the humerus. In cases where the arm is abducted and externally rotated, the shoulder may dislocate, especially in those patients with a limited normal range of external rotation.

Finally, this force may be transmitted through to the clavicle and cause a fracture of the junction of the lateral two-thirds and medial third. The sternoclavicular joint may also dislocate.

Other fractures must also be looked for — not only in the injured arm but elsewhere.

FALLS ON THE OUTSTRETCHED HAND

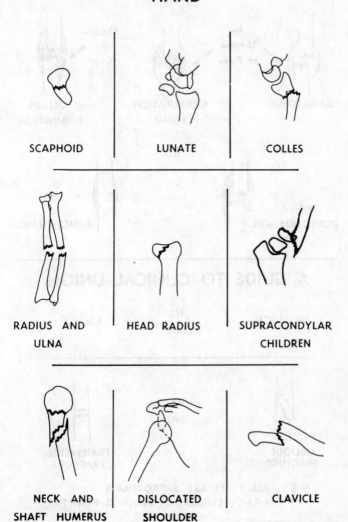

SCAPHOID

LUNATE

COLLES

RADIUS AND ULNA

HEAD RADIUS

SUPRACONDYLAR CHILDREN

NECK AND SHAFT HUMERUS

DISLOCATED SHOULDER

CLAVICLE

HEALING OF FRACTURES

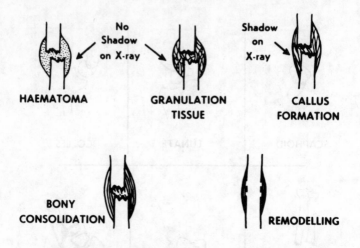

HAEMATOMA → No Shadow on X-ray → **GRANULATION TISSUE** → Shadow on X-ray → **CALLUS FORMATION**

BONY CONSOLIDATION

REMODELLING

A GUIDE TO CLINICAL UNION

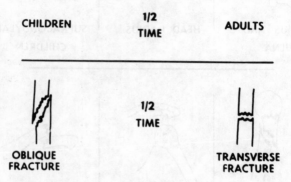

CHILDREN	1/2 TIME	ADULTS

OBLIQUE FRACTURE — 1/2 TIME — **TRANSVERSE FRACTURE**

<u>N.B.</u> ALL TIMES ARE APPROXIMATE
X-RAY + CLINICAL EVIDENCE IS ESSENTIAL

IMMOBILISATION
INJURIES OF THE UPPER LIMBS
APPROXIMATE TIMES

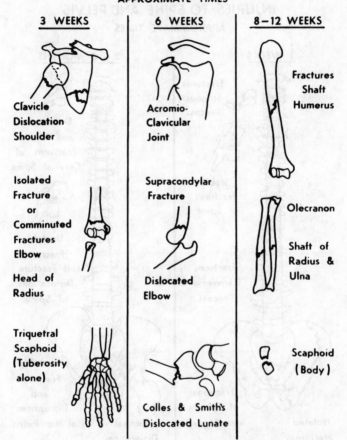

3 WEEKS	6 WEEKS	8–12 WEEKS
Clavicle Dislocation Shoulder	Acromio-Clavicular Joint	Fractures Shaft Humerus
Isolated Fracture or Comminuted Fractures Elbow	Supracondylar Fracture	Olecranon
Head of Radius	Dislocated Elbow	Shaft of Radius & Ulna
Triquetral Scaphoid (Tuberosity alone)	Colles & Smith's Dislocated Lunate	Scaphoid (Body)

NEVER IMMOBILISE SHOULDER OR HAND INJURIES MORE
THAN 3 WEEKS <u>UNLESS</u> IN FUNCTIONAL POSITION

IMMOBILISATION OR NON-WEIGHT-BEARING

INJURIES TO SPINE AND PELVIS
APPROXIMATE TIMES

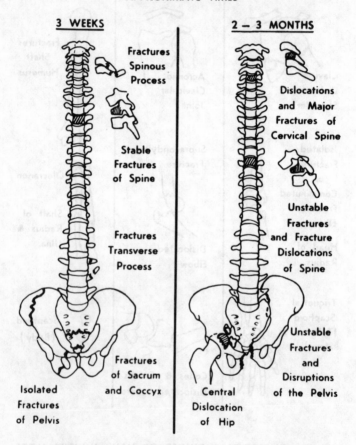

3 WEEKS

Fractures Spinous Process

Stable Fractures of Spine

Fractures Transverse Process

Isolated Fractures of Pelvis

Fractures of Sacrum and Coccyx

2 – 3 MONTHS

Dislocations and Major Fractures of Cervical Spine

Unstable Fractures and Fracture Dislocations of Spine

Central Dislocation of Hip

Unstable Fractures and Disruptions of the Pelvis

TREATMENT OF NEUROLOGICAL AND BLADDER COMPLICATIONS TAKES PRECEDENCE OVER FRACTURES

IMMOBILISATION
INJURIES OF THE LOWER LIMBS
APPROXIMATE TIMES

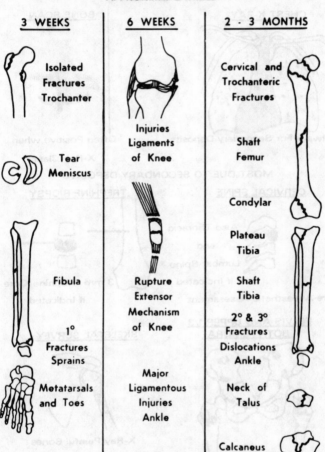

3 WEEKS	6 WEEKS	2 - 3 MONTHS
Isolated Fractures Trochanter	Injuries Ligaments of Knee	Cervical and Trochanteric Fractures
Tear Meniscus		Shaft Femur
		Condylar
Fibula	Rupture Extensor Mechanism of Knee	Plateau Tibia
		Shaft Tibia
1° Fractures Sprains		2° & 3° Fractures Dislocations Ankle
Metatarsals and Toes	Major Ligamentous Injuries Ankle	Neck of Talus
		Calcaneus

NEVER ALLOW WEIGHT BEARING TOO EARLY
EARLY PHYSIOTHERAPY IS ESSENTIAL

PATHOLOGICAL FRACTURES
DIAGNOSIS & PRE-OPERATIVE ASSESSMENT

CHEST X-RAY

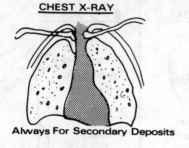

Always For Secondary Deposits

BONE SCAN

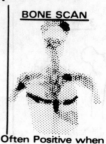

Often Positive when

X-Ray Clear

MOST DUE TO SECONDARY DEPOSITS

CERVICAL SPINE

Also Thoracic

and

Lumbar Spine

if Indicated

Pre-Anaesthetic Assessment

TREPHINE BIOPSY

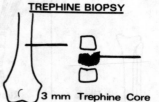

3 mm Trephine Core

if Indicated

PELVIS AND UPPER 1/3 BOTH FEMORA

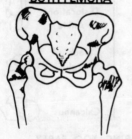

SKELETAL SURVEY

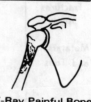

X-Ray Painful Bones

Tomogram if Necessary

ALWAYS COMPLETE PHYSICAL EXAMINATION

AND BLOOD ASSESSMENT PRE-OPERATIVELY

PATHOLOGICAL FRACTURES
TREATMENT

<u>**HUMERUS**</u>

Upper End and Shaft

<u>**HUMERUS**</u>

Lower End

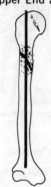

Sling or Collar and Cuff
ONLY if Necessary

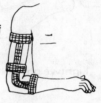

Rush Nail

Skelecast

<u>SHOULDER AND HUMERUS</u>

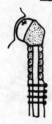

Huckstep Titanium and
Ceramic Shoulder plus
Humeral Replacement
if Necessary

<u>RADIUS AND ULNA</u>

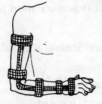

Skelecast   OR   Rush Nail

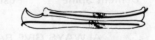

PATHOLOGICAL FRACTURES

TREATMENT

CERVICAL SPINE

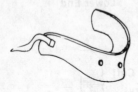

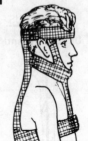

Lightweight Collar   **OR**   **Skelecast Minerva**
(Roman soldier)

THORACIC AND	PELVIS AND
LUMBAR SPINE	ACETABULUM

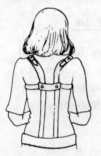

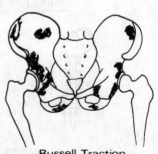

Russell Traction

Taylor Brace   **Crutches as soon as possible**

Cement Spine   **Posterior Stabilization of the Spine**

ALWAYS GIVE RADIOTHERAPY
OR SPECIFIC CHEMOTHERAPY

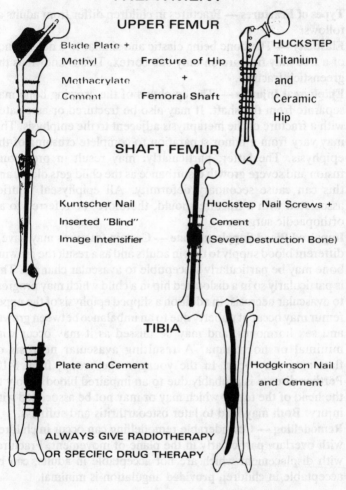

PATHOLOGICAL FRACTURES
TREATMENT

UPPER FEMUR

Blade Plate +
Methyl
Methacrylate
Cement

Fracture of Hip
+
Femoral Shaft

HUCKSTEP
Titanium
and
Ceramic
Hip

SHAFT FEMUR

Kuntscher Nail
Inserted "Blind"
Image Intensifier

Huckstep Nail Screws +
Cement
(Severe Destruction Bone)

TIBIA

Plate and Cement

Hodgkinson Nail
and Cement

ALWAYS GIVE RADIOTHERAPY
OR SPECIFIC DRUG THERAPY

FRACTURES IN CHILDREN

Types of Fractures — Fractures in children differ from adults as follows:

Elasticity — The bone being elastic and similar to a new branch of a tree may fracture on only one cortex. This is known as the greenstick fracture.

Epiphyseal Injuries — The epiphysis of the growing bone may separate from the shaft. It may also be fractured or associated with a fracture of the metaphysis adjacent to the epiphysis. This may vary from a minor separation to complete crushing of the epiphysis. The latter, particularly, may result in premature fusion and severe growth disturbance as the child gets older, and this can cause secondary deformity. All epiphyseal injuries associated with a fracture should, therefore, be referred to an orthopaedic surgeon.

Impaired Blood Supply to Bone — Certain fractures may have a different blood supply to that in adults and as a result the growing bone may be particularly susceptible to avascular changes. This is particularly so in a dislocated hip in a child which may progress to avascular necrosis. In addition a slipped epiphysis of the upper femur may occur at puberty due to an imbalance between growth and sex hormones, and may be missed as it may occur with minimal or no trauma. A resulting avascular necrosis or flattening may ocur. In the younger age group, from 5-10, Perthes disease is probably due to an impaired blood supply to the head of the femur which may or may not be associated with injury. Both may lead to later osteoarthritis and stiffness.

Remodelling — Considerable remodelling can occur in children with overlap, particularly in the plane of movement. Fractures with displacement which are not acceptable in adults, can be acceptable in children **provided** angulation is minimal.

FRACTURES IN CHILDREN

COMMON FRACTURES
GREENSTICK FRACTURES

| FEMUR | TIBIA | RADIUS & ULNA | HUMERUS | CLAVICLE |

SLIPPED EPIPHYSIS
(FRACTURE SEPARATION)

SUPRACONDYLAR
FRACTURE HUMERUS

FEMUR   Lower End   Head
     RADIUS   TIBIA

EPIPHYSEAL DAMAGE
CLASSIFICATION

| Type I | Type II | Type III | Type IV | Type V |

  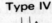 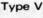

| COMPLETE SEPARATION YOUNG CHILDREN NO FRACTURE EASY REDUCTION GOOD PROGNOSIS | COMMONEST TYPE OLDER CHILDREN EASY REDUCTION GOOD PROGNOSIS | UNCOMMON INTRA-ARTICULAR OPEN REDUCTION USUALLY NECESSARY PROGNOSIS FAIRLY GOOD | INTRA-ARTICULAR OPEN REDUCTION & FIXATION NECESSARY PROGNOSIS USUALLY POOR UNLESS PERFECT REDUCTION | UNCOMMON CRUSHING INJURIES DIAGNOSIS DIFFICULT PROGNOSIS POOR |

SUPRACONDYLAR FRACTURES

A supracondylar fracture of the humerus with displacement in a child is a surgical emergency, as it may cause pressure on the brachial artery or bleeding under the flexor sheath of the forearm with Volkmann's ischaemic contracture. These children must always be admitted to hospital.

STRESS FRACTURES

These are due to repetitive minor injury often from unaccustomed exertion, particularly in the growing child, and are common. They may be misdiagnosed as there may be no history of trauma and the fracture may be very difficult to see until 2 or 3 weeks have elapsed and the callus formation has started to calcify.

The common sites are the tibia, fibula and necks of the metatarsals. A bone scan is a useful diagnostic aid if x-ray is negative.

PRINCIPLES OF TREATMENT

General — Treatment should be based on suspicion, as the diagnosis of the fracture in children may be difficult, particularly if the child is young.

Pain in the knee may be an indication of an early slip of the epiphysis of the hip, and the adolescent child's hip should always be x-rayed and treated on suspicion by non-weight bearing and traction in hospital if necessary.

X-rays of the epiphyses and bones in the child may be confusing, particularly around the elbow. If in doubt, the other side should be x-rayed in **exactly** the same position, and a comparision made.

FRACTURES IN CHILDREN
DIAGNOSIS

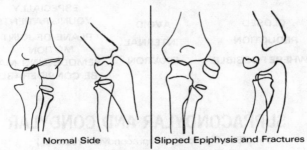

Normal Side | Slipped Epiphysis and Fractures

X-RAY OPPOSITE SIDE IN JOINT INJURIES

EXAMINATION

Look for Infection
Mimicking Fracture

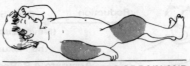

LOOK FOR OTHER INJURIES AND CAUSES OF PAIN AND OR PARALYSIS

BABIES

Look for
Battered Baby Syndrome
Complete Systematic
Examination
Including Chest
and Abdomen
Always Admit to
Hospital
and Photograph

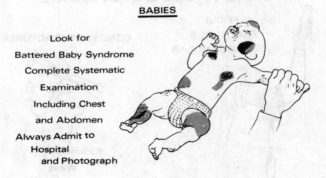

FRACTURES IN CHILDREN
PRINCIPLES OF TREATMENT

CLOSED
REDUCTION
WHERE POSSIBLE

AVOID
INTERNAL
FIXATION

ESPECIALLY
YOUNG PATIENTS
PLANE OF JOINT
MOTION
REMODELLING MAY
BE CONSIDERABLE

SUPRACONDYLAR AND CONDYLAR
(Also See Section on Supracondylar Fractures)

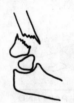

Reduction →

Padded
Back Slab
(Never Encircle
the Flexure)
Accurate A.P. Reduction

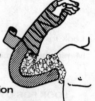

CARE VASCULAR DAMAGE

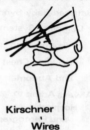

DIFFICULT
FRACTURES
SUPRACONDLAR

CONDYLAR FRACTURES

Kirschner
Wires

FRACTURES IN CHILDREN

NECK FEMUR
Always Internally Fix

SHAFT FEMUR
15 Kg. Weight of Baby

Up to 1cm Shortening

Acceptable Due to Compensatory Overgrowth

Knee Supported in Slight Flexion

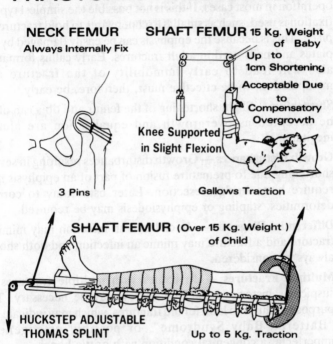

3 Pins

Gallows Traction

SHAFT FEMUR (Over 15 Kg. Weight) of Child

HUCKSTEP ADJUSTABLE THOMAS SPLINT

Up to 5 Kg. Traction
(approximately ½ Kg./Year of Age)

RADIUS AND ULNA

Greenstick Fractures of Wrist Common

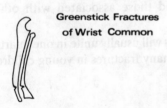

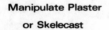

Manipulate Plaster or Skelecast

TIBIA AND FIBULA

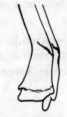

Manipulate Plaster or Skelecast

Avoidance of Operation — Treatment should be without operation in most cases. If this is not possible the simplest type of fixation is used, such as small Kirschner wires to hold fractures in place. This is because the epiphysis can be easily damaged by the plates and nails used in adult fractures. Early callus formation also will lead to early immobility of the fracture and manipulation, to be effective must, therefore, be early.

Shortening — Slight shortening of the femur and tibia can often be accepted as overgrowth and equalization are almost inevitable.

Growth Disturbances — Growth disturbances resulting in severe shortening due to premature fusion of part of an epiphysis may require bone bridge resection. Later osteotomy to correct deformities, stapling or epiphysiodesis may be required.

Differential Diagnosis — In children an infection may mimic a fracture and a fracture may mimic an infection and both should always be considered.

Multiple Fractures — In babies with multiple fractures or suspicious histories a skeletal survey may be necessary. The purpose of this is to look for old fractures, which may indicate the "Battered Baby Syndrome", or possibly osteogenesis imperfecta, a congenital condition with brittle bones.

Internal Injuries — Care in children should be especially exercised to avoid missing internal injuries, particularly of the head, chest and abdomen and those associated with other fractures.

Healing — In children, fractures will usually unite in one quarter to half the time of adults and many fractures in young children are united in 3 weeks.

FRACTURES IN CHILDREN
COMPLICATIONS

OVERGROWTH

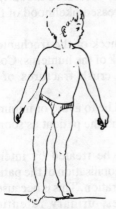

Fractures Often Stimulate
Overgrowth of 1-2cm

Avoid Overdistracting Fractures
in Children

MALUNION

Angulation
Must be
Corrected

SHORTENING

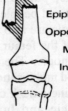

Epiphysiodesis
Opposite Side
May be
Indicated

GROWTH DISTURBANCES

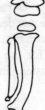

Varus or Valgus
Due to Epiphyseal
Damage

AVASCULAR NECROSIS

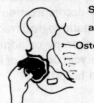

Stiffness
and Late
Osteoarthritis

FRACTURES IN OLD PEOPLE

There are certain fractures which are particularly common in old people, and this is partly due to senile osteoporosis. Other factors include diminished muscle tone, decreased mobility of joint and spine due to arthritis and increased likelihood of falls due to a variety of causes.

Common fractures are those of the neck or the trochanteric region of the femur, fractures of the neck of the humerus, Colles fractures of the wrist and multiple crush fractures of an osteoporotic spine.

The principle of the treatment should be to avoid or minimise hospitalisation and to mobilise joints and the patient as soon as possible.

Fractures of the hip should **always** be treated by internal fixation as soon as possible, with early mobilisation of the patient out of bed **within** a day or two of the operation. This is because of the complications of pressure sores, urinary retention, bronchopneumonia, contractures of joints, deep vein thrombosis, pulmonary embolus and mental disturbance common in old people left in bed for long periods.

Old people are also particularly likely to sustain **pathological** fractures of the femur and humerus due to secondary deposits from carcinoma. The principle here should be early internal fixation and mobilisation, wherever possible. In fractures of the cervical spine a neck collar, plus radiotherapy, is indicated. In the thoracic and lumbar spine a lightweight brace and radiotherapy will often allow early mobility. Occasionally emergency decompression of the spine may be needed. After fixation of pathological fractures many patients can return home after radiotherapy or adjuvant chemotherapy for the last few months, or year or two, of life rather than languishing in nursing homes and hospitals.

COMMON FRACTURES IN OLD PEOPLE

COLLES FRACTURE

SHOULDER FRACTURE OR DISLOCATION

FEMUR NECK OR TROCHANTER

PRINCIPLES
{
EARLY MOBILISATION

AVOID
{
Joint Stiffness
Pressure Sores
Bladder & Lung
Complications
}
}

Think of the **WHOLE** Patient

FRACTURES DUE TO FALLS FROM A HEIGHT

FRACTURE SPINE

CENTRAL DISLOCATION OF HIP

FRACTURE CALCANEUS

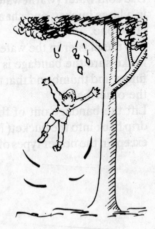

PLASTER OF PARIS TECHNIQUE

TYPES OF PLASTER BANDAGE

Plaster bandages come in the following sizes: 5, 7.5, 10 and 15cm suitable for hands and arms, 10cm and 15cm suitable for legs and for plaster back slabs, hip spicas and plaster jackets. This plaster hardens completely in 24 to 48 hours, but is fairly strong in 1 to 2 hours and firm in about 5 minutes, depending on the plaster and the temperature of the water. There are newer plasters which are water resistant and which do not drip and lose plaster into the bucket, and these should be used where possible.

APPLICATION OF PLASTER BANDAGES

It is important that plaster bandages are applied quickly and well if pressure sores and other complications are to be avoided. The following points are important:-

DIPPING OF THE PLASTER

1. Use cold water (warm water if more rapid setting is required) in a large bucket, and change the water if the plaster is a very large one.
2. Dip the plaster in the water until the bubbles stop appearing. Make sure the bandage is held firmly in the middle with the finger and thumb and that the edge of the bandage is held with the other hand.
3. Lift the bandage out of the water and let the surplus water drip back into the bucket(**NOT** on the floor!). Do **not** squeeze **except** in the newer types of plaster which drip relatively little.

PLASTER OF PARIS
EQUIPMENT

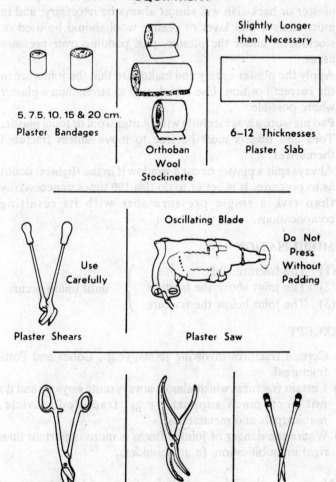

5, 7.5, 10, 15 & 20 cm.
Plaster Bandages

Slightly Longer than Necessary

Orthoban Wool Stockinette

6-12 Thicknesses Plaster Slab

Use Carefully

Plaster Shears

Oscillating Blade

Do Not Press Without Padding

Plaster Saw

Plaster Scissors

Plaster Benders

Plaster Openers

APPLYING THE PLASTER

1. In acute fractures requiring manipulations, a well **padded** plaster or back-slab will almost always be necessary, and in most cases a thin layer of plaster wool should be used or stockinette under the plaster, plus padding over pressure areas.
2. Apply the plaster evenly and make sure that the joints are in the correct position. Use a back-slab to strengthen a plaster where possible.
3. Pad pressure areas carefully with plaster wool or foam plastic. Toes and fingers must be free to move unless fractured themselves.
4. Always split a plaster or cut a window if in the slightest doubt as to pressure. It is better to do this **100** times unnecessarily than risk a single pressure sore with its resulting complications.

IMMOBILISATION

(1) The fracture site
(2) The joint above the fracture $\Big\}$ until union occurs
(3) The joint below the fracture

EXCEPT

(a) Certain fractures involving joints, (e.g., Colles and Potts fractures).
(b) Certain fractures which almost always unite anyway and do not need much support, (e.g., fractured clavicle, metacarpals and metatarsals).
(c) Where the danger of joint stiffness is more important than rigid immobilisation, (e.g., shoulder).

Always use aluminium splints for finger and wrist injuries, where possible, and **skelecasts** in all cases where manipulation is not necessary.

PLASTER OF PARIS
TECHNIQUE

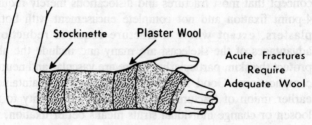

Stockinette

Plaster Wool

Acute Fractures
Require
Adequate Wool

Padding

Wait
Until
Bubbles
Cease

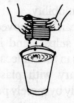

Do Not
Squeeze
Allow to
Drip

Dipping Plaster

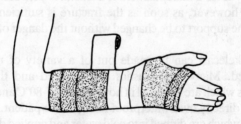

Application of Plaster
Complete Plaster
Slab Held with Cotton Bandage

SKELECASTS

The skelecast is a simple concept of lightweight fixation of the limbs and trunk invented by the author in 1966. It is based on the concept that most fractures and dislocations merely require 3 or 4-point fixation and not complete encasement with hot, heavy plasters, **except** where a fracture requires reduction. The advantages of the skelecast are many and include the ability to protect the skin, particularly if there are vascular and neurological complications. Good skin and muscle tone is maintained with earlier union of fractures in most cases. The ability to tighten, loosen or change individual struts means better fixation, in most cases, than with complete encasement in plaster.

The lightness of weight and the waterproof nature of the support enables patients to have daily showers, to swim and often to return to work. Hinges can be incorporated in the knee and elbow to allow for even better mobility.

The supports can be removed easily by simply cutting through the struts with "tin snips", and in most cases, x-rays can be taken through the gaps in the skelecast without removing the skelecast, as is often necessary with plaster. In acute fractures oedema is controlled initially by merely putting a little wool and crepe bandage round the limb between the struts until the swelling has settled.

Skelecasts are **not** usually indicated where a complete wrap is necessary after a manipulation of a fracture. The skelecast can be applied, however, as soon as the fracture is sufficiently stable to enable the support to be changed without the danger of the fracture slipping.

The skelecast can be made out of a variety of materials, as illustrated. Many new plastics can be used and these include materials which are softened in hot water at 65-80°C and are applied as struts directly over waterproof lining to the patient. Waterproof plasters, which are dipped into cold water and applied directly to the patient in the form of struts, can also be used, as well as polyester resin, and a light sensitive resin. Newer materials are constantly being developed and the one most suited and available, should be used.

SKELECASTS

TECHNIQUE FOR APPLICATION
OF THERMOPLASTICS

Waterproof
Lining or Plastic
Foam

Thermoplastic
65 80°C

Cut Strips of Thermoplastic
and Lining into Short Strips,
enough for Overlap of 1 - 2cm.

TECHNIQUE OF CYLINDER
SKELECASTS

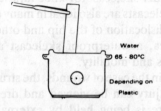

Water
65 - 80°C

Depending on
Plastic

Dip Thermoplastic Briefly into Water

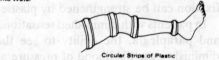

Waterproof Lining

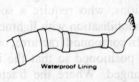

Circular Strips of Plastic

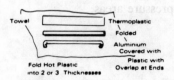

Towel

Thermoplastic
Folded
Aluminium
Covered with
Plastic with
Overlap at Ends

Fold Hot Plastic
into 2 or 3 Thicknesses

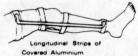

Longitudinal Strips of
Covered Aluminium

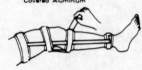

Further Circular Strips

The longitudinal struts of the skelecasts are usually strengthened with thin aluminium struts covered by one or two layers of the plastic or material used in the manufacture of the support. The detail of the exact type of plastic or metal used is unimportant, provided that good rigid fixation is obtained, the support is waterproof and strong, and the points of contact between the struts are properly moulded and strengthened if necessary.

The scaphoid skelecast is ideal. Other suitable indications include above-elbow skelecast for the radius and ulna after internal fixation of fractures, and the Colles type support for fractures of the wrist **not requiring** manipulation.

In the lower limb the cylinder skelecast for knee injuries and above and below the knee skelecasts are also ideal in many cases. In children with congenital dislocation of the hip and other hip lesions, who require a spica, a waterproof skelecast allows immobilisation with lightness and mobility.

In compound fractures, or in the case of wounds, the struts can be positioned so that the injury can be viewed and dressings changed. Where the fracture is being held by external pins fixation can be strengthened by plastic struts.

In patients with diminished sensation, such as in nerve injuries and paraplegia, the ability to see the skin under the struts diminishes the likelihood of pressure areas.

THERMOPLASTIC SKELECAST

Thermoplastic Bandage ⟶ Apply Strips
in Hot Water 60 - 80° C over Foam Padding

LIGHTCAST SKELECAST

Lightcast Bandage   Light Source   Hardens 15 secs
1''-6'' Bandages + 3.200 - 4.000 A ▸ Cures 3 minutes

POLYESTER RESIN SKELECAST

Polyester Resin Putty + Hardener ▸ Impregnate Glass Fibre Tape

SKELECAST JACKET

All Skelecasts - Use Waterproof
Polythylene or Plastazote
between Skelecast and Skin
Use ¼inch and ½inch Aluminium Strips
covered in Thermoplastic

1 Front Strut for Women ⎤ Strengthen Joints with
2 Front Struts for Men ⎦ Extra Resin

THERMOPLASTIC

Easily Adjustable and Easily Repaired
Repair with Epoxy Resin or Thermoplastic

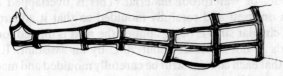

Remove with Plaster Shears or Plaster Saw

In the operating theatre, in patients having operations such as a patellectomy, screwing of an ankle fracture or internal fixation of fractures of the radius and ulna, lower humerus or olecranon, a plaster back-slab over wool is applied for about 3 days until the suction drain has been removed and the post-operative oedema has diminished. It is a simple matter then for the skelecast to be applied. Many thousands of skelecasts have been applied since this concept was first developed in 1966, and the average time of union of fractures is approximately 2/3rds of the equivalent time in complete plaster encasement. This is presumably due to the better tone of muscles, the increased use of the limb and the good skin texture in limbs supported by skelecasts. In addition, joints immobilised with skelecasts, even **without** a hinge, rapidly regain their movement after removal of the skelecast, which is very different from plaster immobilisation.

METHOD OF APPLICATION

The method of application of a skelecast is illustrated, and is simple once the technique is mastered. It often takes longer to apply than a simple complete wrap of plaster or synthetic material, but its many advantages more than compensate for this. Patients who have once experienced a skelecast will not return to plaster fixation.

Firstly, thin strips of waterproof lining one layer of thickness are put round the arm or leg, as illustrated, and overlapped slightly and held in place with small strips of tape. These are then covered with about 2 or 3 thicknesses of hot thermo-plastic or other plastic, or waterproof material. This is overlapped by about 3cm on itself and carefully moulded so that it adheres. While one circular strut is being applied the next is dipped for a few seconds in hot water at about 70°C by an assistant. It is important that each circular strut be carefully moulded and made to adhere to itself before the next one is applied. It is also useful to have all the circular and longitudinal struts cut to the right length from 5 or 7.5cm wide plastic, before they are dipped.

SKELECASTS
UPPER LIMB

Crepe Bandage
Over Wool for
Oedema

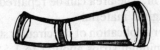

COLLES

Patients can
Bathe and Swim
Cast is Waterproof
and Light

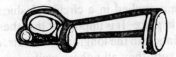

SCAPHOID

Flexion at Elbow
Adjustable by
Cutting Struts and
Repairing if Necessary

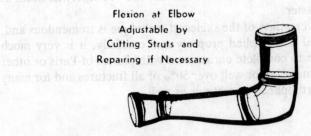

ABOVE ELBOW

It is then a simple matter to dip each one in turn in the hot water, lay it on a towel to fold it on itself 2 or 3 times and then apply it directly over the lining. Gloves are not necessary due to the low conductivity of the plastic. If any of the circular struts are too loose or too tight they can be easily cut or opened out or closed in. The area can be repaired with an epoxy resin glue or the original material.

After application of the circular strut, 2 or 3 longitudinal struts of aluminium strips about 1 to 1.5 cm in diameter are covered with a layer of thermo-plastic. The aluminium strip is cut to exactly the correct length and is overlapped by about 1cm at each end by the plastic which can then be turned over on to the circular strut for added fixation, as illustrated. Each end of the longitudial strut can be dipped in hot water for a few seconds to soften this again before applying. Extra strips of thermo-plastic are then applied in a circular fashion to hold the longitudinal struts in place. It is important that these are carefully moulded at the joints with the longitudinal struts, and to the circular struts to make sure they all adhere well.

If for any reason a strut needs to be removed, for x-ray or for radiotherapy, this can be easily done and it can be repositioned. In the case of elbows or knees a hinge can be inserted to allow for flexion of the joint, provided the last 20-30 degrees of extension is prevented. Rotation at the fracture site will otherwise occur as with plaster.

The versatility of the skelecast technique is tremendous and, provided it is applied properly and carefully, it is very much superior to complete encasement with plaster-of-Paris or other plastic material for well over 50% of all fractures and for many other orthopaedic conditions as well.

SKELECASTS

LOWER LIMB

Position of Strips Adjustable
for Ease of Dressings

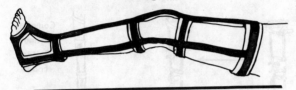

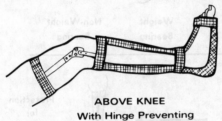

Adjustable
For
Tightness

ABOVE KNEE
With Hinge Preventing
Last 20° of Extension

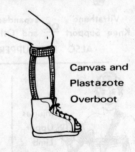

Canvas and
Plastazote
Overboot

BELOW KNEE WEIGHT-BEARING

Alternatively Complete Lightcast will Allow Full
Weight - bearing

ORTHOPAEDIC SPLINTS
CALIPERS AND SUPPORTS

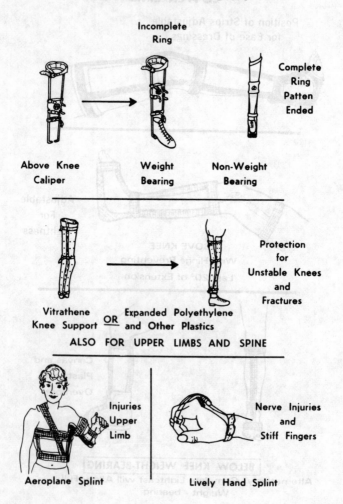

Incomplete Ring

Complete Ring Patten Ended

Above Knee Caliper

Weight Bearing

Non-Weight Bearing

Vitrathene Knee Support OR Expanded Polyethylene and Other Plastics

Protection for Unstable Knees and Fractures

ALSO FOR UPPER LIMBS AND SPINE

Injuries Upper Limb

Aeroplane Splint

Nerve Injuries and Stiff Fingers

Lively Hand Splint

ORTHOPAEDIC TABLE

Abduct Legs
Sufficiently

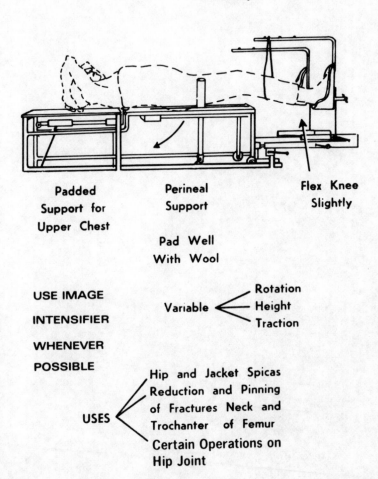

Padded
Support for
Upper Chest

Perineal
Support

Flex Knee
Slightly

Pad Well
With Wool

USE IMAGE
INTENSIFIER
WHENEVER
POSSIBLE

Variable ⟨ Rotation
Height
Traction

USES ⟨ Hip and Jacket Spicas
Reduction and Pinning
of Fractures Neck and
Trochanter of Femur
Certain Operations on
Hip Joint

ORTHOPAEDIC TABLE

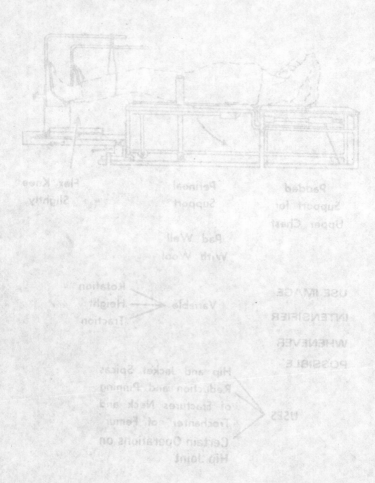

Abduct Legs
Sufficiently

Flex Knee
Slightly

Perineal
Support

Padded
Support for
Upper Chest

Pad Well
With Wool

Rotation
Variable — Height
Traction

USE IMAGE
INTENSIFIER
WHENEVER
POSSIBLE

Hip and Jacket Spicas
Reduction and Pinning
of Fractures Neck and
Trochanter of Femur
Certain Operations on
Hip Joint

USES

UPPER LIMB

FINGERS — MINOR INJURIES

DISLOCATED FINGER

(1) **Reduce** by a firm pull with elastoplast on the fingers to obtain a purchase. A digital nerve block can be used in adults, a general anaesthetic in children and sometimes **no** anaesthetic in suitable patients.

(2) The finger should be held reduced for 1-3 weeks in **slight flexion** by a finger splint of padded aluminium, as illustrated. This is important to diminish the likelihood of stiffness and pain, which is common.

(3) Energetic active exercises should be given to regain movements, and the joint supported with elastoplast to prevent swelling for 2 or 3 weeks after splint is removed.

FRACTURE OF THE MIDDLE OR DISTAL PHALANX

(1) **Reduce** if necessary.

(2) **Hold** reduced for 3 weeks in **slight flexion** by a padded aluminium finger splint, as illustrated.

(3) **Then** energetic active exercises, irrespective of the position of the fracture. Support also with elastoplast if necessary for 2 or 3 weeks.

FRACTURE OF THE PROXIMAL PHALANX

(1) Reduce only if necessary. It is important to correct mal-rotation.

(2) **Hold** reduced for 2 to 3 weeks with the metacarpophalangeal joint **well flexed** by a padded aluminium splint extending into the palm, as illustrated.

(3) **Then** energetic active exercises, irrespective of the position of the fracture. Support by elastoplast may also be helpful.

Alternatively 2 or 3 layers of elastoplast, rather than an aluminium splint, can be used.

FINGER INJURIES

DISLOCATED FINGERS

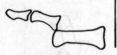 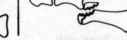

WITHOUT FRACTURE   **WITH FRACTURE**   **WITH RUPTURED TENDON**

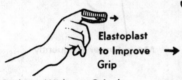 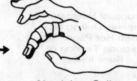

Elastoplast to Improve Grip →

Reduce Without G.A. by Firm Pull and Flexion

Aluminium Splint
(S) For 1—3 Weeks
for Ruptured Tendon

Always Use Padded Aluminium Strip if Available

FRACTURE MIDDLE OR DISTAL PHALANX

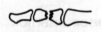 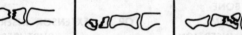 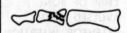

MIDDLE PHALANX   **DISTAL PHALANX**   **INVOLVING JOINT**

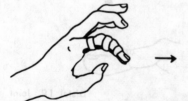

→ REDUCE ONLY IF MUCH DISPLACEMENT IMMOBILISE FOR 1—3 WEEKS EARLY MOVEMENTS

INTERNAL FIXATION IF NECESSARY IF JOINT INVOLVED

FINGER INJURIES

SPRAINED and BRUISED FINGERS

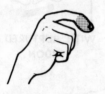

Strap with Elastoplast (1 Week) →

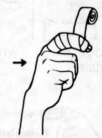

Tip of Finger Visible

Subungual Haematoma Requires Drilling Nail or Red Hot Paper Clip Exclude Tendon or Bone Injury

Move Finger Frequently

MALLET FINGER

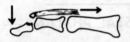 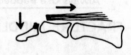

CHIP OF BONE AVULSED FROM EXTENSOR INSERTION **OR** EXTENSOR INSERTION RUPTURED

MALLET FINGER SPLINT FOR 4 WEEKS ONLY 50% RECOVER MINIMAL DISABILITY

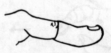

Distal I.P. Joint Hyperextended

FINGER INJURIES

FRACTURE OF PROXIMAL PHALANX

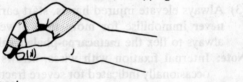

NOT INVOLVING JOINT   **INVOLVING JOINT**

REDUCE IF NECESSARY

THEN

Screw or Kirschner Wire
ONLY
for Displacement into Joint

MOST CASES

Padded Aluminium Front Splint Held by Strapping

Metacarpo-Phalangeal
Joint Well Flexed

IMMOBILISE FOR 1—3 WEEKS
THEN
ENERGETIC ACTIVE EXERCISES

FINGERS — MAJOR INJURIES

SEVERAL FRACTURES OF THE FINGERS

(1) **Reduce if necessary.** Closed reduction is usually sufficient, but open reduction with Kirschner wire fixation may occasionally be necessary.

(2) **Hold** reduced with a pad of wool in the palm and a bandage to hold metacarpo-phalangeal joints well flexed and interphalangeal joints near extension.

(3) Energetic active exercises after 3 weeks, irrespective of the position of the fractures.

COMPOUND FRACTURES OF THE FINGERS

(1) **Reduce** if possible, and close wounds if clean.

(2) **Hold** reduced as for simple fractures.

(3) **Then** energetic active exercises.

STIFF OR BADLY INFECTED FINGERS

(1) Always preserve as much **thumb** as possible **irrespective** of stiffness or infection.

(2) Always amputate **other** fingers **early,** if stiff or badly infected. An amputated finger is always preferable to a stiff and useless hand.

(3) Always elevate injured hands, start early movements, and **never** immobilise for more than 3 weeks. **REMEMBER** always to flex the **metacarpo-phalangeal** joints **well.**

Note: Internal fixation with wires, screws or small plates is occasionally indicated for severe fractures or dislocations of fingers where **non-**operative measures have failed, especially in joint involvement.

ALUMINIUM COCK UP SPLINT

A padded aluminium front splint with the wrist dorsiflexed is useful for many hand, wrist and lower forearm injuries as either an emergency or definitive support.

FINGER INJURIES

SEVERE HAND INJURIES

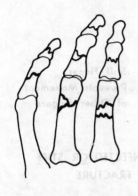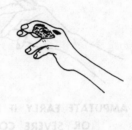

SEVERAL FRACTURES   COMPOUND FRACTURES

REDUCE IF BADLY
DISPLACED

INTERNAL FIXATION IF NECESSARY

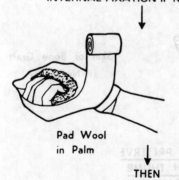

Pad Wool
in Palm

Hold Reduced with
Crepe Bandage
1—3 Weeks
MP Joints
Well Flexed

THEN

ENERGETIC ACTIVE EXERCISES

FINGER INJURIES

STIFF OR BADLY INFECTED FINGERS

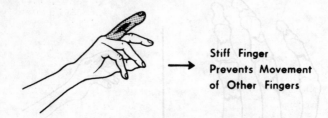

Stiff Finger
Prevents Movement
of Other Fingers

**AMPUTATE EARLY IF BADLY INFECTED <u>OR</u> STIFF
<u>OR</u> SEVERE COMPOUND FRACTURE**

STIFF OR BADLY INFECTED THUMB

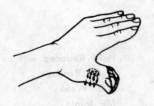

Skin or Bone Graft
if Necessary

**<u>ALWAYS PRESERVE
AS MUCH THUMB
AS POSSIBLE</u>**

FINGER INJURIES

COMPLICATIONS

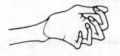

→ ALWAYS IMMOBILISE
FINGERS IN
SLIGHT FLEXION
PLUS
METACARPOPHALANGEAL
JOINTS IN 90° FLEXION

STIFF FINGERS
Especially Extended
Metacarpo-Phalangeal
Joints

GIVE EARLY ACTIVE
MOVEMENTS

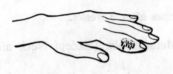

→ PROPHYLACTIC
CHEMOTHERAPY
EARLY SURGERY
IMMOBILISATION
IN FLEXION
M.P.JOINTS

**INFECTION AND
OSTEOMYELITIS**

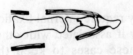

→ SUTURE EXTENSOR TENDONS

→ 2nd STAGE TENDON GRAFT
FOR FLEXOR TENDONS
IN FLEXOR SHEATH

TENDON DAMAGE

FRACTURES OF THE METACARPALS

Classification:
1. Fracture dislocation of base of first metacarpal (Bennett's)
2. Fracture of neck of metacarpal
3. All other fractures of metacarpals.

Fracture of Neck of Metacarpal:
(a) Reduce only in severe angulation by flexing the proximal phalanx.
(b) **Hold** reduced for 2-3 weeks with a padded aluminium **front** splint with the metacarpo-phalangeal joint **flexed** to a right angle if possible. An aluminium front splint made out of a T splint can, however, be a useful support in fractures of the neck of the 5th metacarpal. A simple aluminium front splint or a crepe bandage may be sufficient for most fractures with minimal displacement.
(c) **Then energetic active exercises after 3 weeks.**

All Other Fractures of the Metacarpals: (Except Neck and Bennett's)
(a) Reduction is **not** usually required, except in **severe** cases where a Kirschner wire may be used.
(b) **Hold** for 2 — 3 weeks in an aluminium cock-up splint. A crepe bandage, however, is all that is required for minor cases. A collar and cuff sling should be used for the first few days to diminish swelling.
(c) **Then** energetic active exercises.

Badly Displaced Fractures: These may require internal fixation with wires or small plates, especially if associated with other injuries. It is important in all these cases to keep the metacarpo-phalangeal joints well flexed. They should not be immobilised for more than 3 weeks. Early active assisted exercises are essential as soon as the fracture has healed.

FRACTURES OF THE METACARPALS

ALL FRACTURES <u>EXCEPT</u> 1st METACARPAL AND NECKS 2nd – 5th

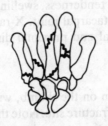

IMMOBILISATION

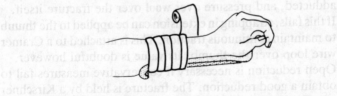

CREPE BANDAGE ALONE OR LIGHTWEIGHT ALUMINIUM SPLINT

FOR 2–3 WEEKS OCCASIONALLY COLLES PLASTER

NOTE : PLASTER SELDOM REQUIRED

POST–REDUCTION

Remove support in 2-3 Weeks

Then Energetic Active Exercises

BENNETT'S FRACTURE

Fracture Dislocation Of Base Of First Carpo-Metacarpal Joint: In this fracture the base of the first metacarpal has a fracture extending into the joint. It is essential that this fracture be reduced properly, as the mobility of the thumb is largely dependent on the joint.

Diagnosis — There is tenderness, swelling and loss of movement of the first carpo-metacarpal joint. X-ray shows a fracture into the joint, with lateral and proximal displacement of the first metacarpal.

Treatment:
1. **Reduce** by traction on the thumb, with **full adduction** and pressure over the fracture site. Note that in the past abduction rather than adduction was advocated, but in many cases adduction produces a better reduction.
2. **Hold reduced** for 4 weeks in complete "scaphoid" type plaster extending to the interphalangeal joint, with the thumb fully adducted, and pressure over **wool** over the fracture itself.
3. If this fails, strapping in extension can be applied to the thumb to maintain continuous traction. This is attached to a Cramer wire loop over the thumb. Its value is doubtful however.
4. Open reduction is necessary if conservative measures fail to obtain a good reduction. The fracture is held by a Kirschner wire or screw until united.
5. Energetic **active** exercises are essential after the plaster is removed. Elastoplast strapping of the joint for about a week is also beneficial.

Complications — Stiffness, pain and osteoarthritis may ensue if reduction has been incomplete, or if physiotherapy has not been given after the plaster is removed.

Scaphoid
Lunate
Triquetral
Trapezius, Trapezoid, capatate &
175
                                        itamate

FRACTURES OF THE METACARPALS

FRACTURE DISLOCATION BASE 1st METACARPAL
BENNETT'S FRACTURE

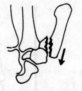

REDUCTION | IMMOBILISATION

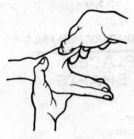

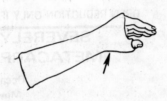

Traction, Adduction,
Pressure Over Base
1st Metacarpal.

**ACCURATE REDUCTION
ESSENTIAL**

Pressure over
Fracture Site
Padded

Plaster to
Interphalangeal
Joint

**NEW TREATMENT
THUMB IN <u>ADDUCTION</u>**

NOTE- OLDER TYPE TREATMENT REQUIRED
THUMB ABDUCTED

POST—REDUCTION

**Remove Plaster in 4 Weeks
<u>Then</u>
Energetic Active Exercises**

FRACTURES OF THE METACARPALS

FAILED REDUCTION OF BENNETT'S FRACTURE

ACCEPT MINOR DISPLACEMENT IN MOST PATIENTS

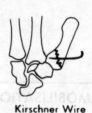

Kirschner Wire

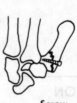

Screw

OPEN REDUCTION ONLY IF CLOSED REDUCTION FAILS

SEVERELY DISPLACED METACARPAL SHAFTS

Occasionally
May Require
INTRAMEDULLARY
Kirschner Wire or Plate

MULTIPLE COMPOUND FRACTURES OF METACARPALS

AS FOR MULTIPLE INJURIES OF HAND

FRACTURES OF THE METACARPALS

FRACTURE NECK METACARPAL

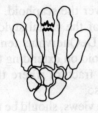

REDUCTION

ONLY IN SEVERE ANGULATION

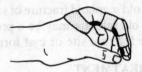

Flex Proximal
Phalanx and
Push Back

1.5 cm Padded Aluminium
Front Splint from
Distal Phalanx to Mid-Palm
for 2-3 Weeks
in 90° Flexion

POST—REDUCTION

Remove Support in 2-3 Weeks

Then

Energetic Active Exercises

SCAPHOID FRACTURE

DIAGNOSIS

This is initially by tenderness over the anatomical snuff box and NOT by x-ray. Upward pressure on the second or third metacarpals may also cause pain over the scaphoid. The main differential diagnosis is a fracture of the radial styloid, which gives tenderness more proximally, DeQuervains tenosynovitis which gives pain over the radial styloid on extending the thumb against resistance, and a Bennett's fracture where the pain is more distal over the metacarpal base.

X-rays, always **including** 2 oblique views, should be taken, but they may sometimes show nothing in the first 3 weeks. "Sprained wrist" is uncommon and is often due to a missed fractured scaphoid. An ununited scaphoid is always very difficult to treat properly and avascular changes in the proximal fragment can ruin a wrist joint. All fractures of the scaphoid must therefore be treated on **suspicion.** Do **not,** however, immobilise unnecessarily an old scaphoid fracture of several months duration. Evidence of an **old** fracture may be a previous history of injury, sclerosis at the fracture site or cyst formation on x-ray.

TREATMENT

Scaphoid Fracture Confirmed On X-Ray — Treatment is a scaphoid plaster or a skelecast left on for 8 weeks. The wrist is then re-examined and re-x-rayed.

If the anatomical snuff box is still tender then, or the x-ray does **not** show trabeculae across the fracture site, another scaphoid plaster or skelecast should be applied for a further 4 weeks before removal and re-x-rayed. **Always** use a skelecast if possible. This need **not** be applied on the day the patient is seen, and a simple aluminium splint can be given safely for about 3 days prior to a skelecast.

FRACTURES OF THE SCAPHOID

WAIST **PROXIMAL POLE** **TUBEROSITY**

CAUSE

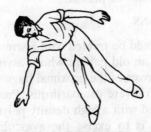

FALL ON THE OUTSTRETCHED HAND

DIAGNOSIS

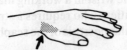

Tender in Anatomical
Snuff Box

Always OBLIQUE X-rays of
Wrist as well as A/P and
Lateral

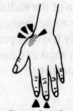

Pain Over Scaphoid on
Pushing on 2nd or
3rd Fingers

If there is non-union after 3 months in an **old** patient the position is either accepted, or the patient treated with a scaphoid splint and the wrist mobilised by physiotherapy. Otherwise a stiff wrist may result. There is also a place for internal fixation with a screw in scaphoid fractures with displacement in the acute stages. In those that have progressed to non-union with an avascular proximal fragment, screw fixation with bone graft, may be indicated, or a prosthetic replacement.

Suspected Scaphoid Fracture - (Not seen initially on x-ray). If there is pain in the anatomical snuff box after an injury, the wrist should be put into a scaphoid support. This is removed at 3 weeks for further x-rays. If a fracture is seen it is treated as above.

Fractures of the Tuberosity of the Scaphoidd - These have a good blood supply and heal well in 3 weeks in a scaphoid, or even a Colles type skelecast or plaster.

COMPLICATIONS

Non-union should be treated with a screw and bone graft, or left untreated in an old patient who is asymptomatic.

Avascular necrosis of the proximal fragment may destroy the wrist and lead to severe osteoarthritis. Prosthetic replacement can be considered with a high density polyethylene prosthesis. The alternative is to excise the avascular fragment or the proximal row of the carpal bones. Both procedures, however, are relatively unsatisfactory and may lead to a painful stiff wrist. Excision of the radial styloid is a fairly small procedure and has a place in some cases. Arthrodesis of the wrist in a working man is probably the best procedure in the patient who requires a strong painless wrist and has a painful avascular necrosis of the scaphoid or osteoarthritis.

FRACTURES OF THE SCAPHOID

TREATMENT
USE SKELECAST IF AVAILABLE

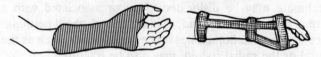

ALWAYS TREAT ON SUSPICION EVEN IF NO FRACTURE SEEN
Immobilise for 8 weeks Initially and THEN X-ray
Put back into Splint if Still Ununited.
Re-X-ray out of Plaster at 3 weeks if Diagnosis is Unconfirmed

EXCEPTIONS TO ABOVE

FRACTURE OF TUBEROSITY - 3 weeks ONLY in Colles Plaster
OLD PEOPLE — Decrease Time of Immobilisation

COMPLICATIONS

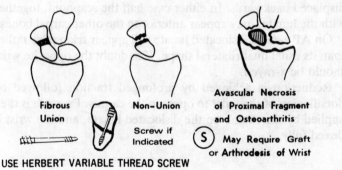

Fibrous
Union

Non-Union

Screw if
Indicated

Avascular Necrosis
of Proximal Fragment
and Osteoarthritis

(S) May Require Graft
or Arthrodesis of Wrist

USE HERBERT VARIABLE THREAD SCREW

DISLOCATION OF THE LUNATE

Dislocation of the lunate is a surgical emergency and the method of dislocation and management is illustrated.

The lunate may be dislocated alone or associated with a fracture of half of the scaphoid, as in the transcaphoid perilunar fracture dislocation. Sometimes other carpal bones, such as the triquetral or the radial styloid, may also be fractured.

In dislocation alone the lunate may be displaced forwards and the wrist may stay intact, or the lunate may be left in place and the whole wrist and carpal bone displaced backwards. The most important complication, particularly with a forward dislocation of the lunate, is pressure of the lunate on the median nerve.

Clinically the wrist is very swollen and painful, with limitation of movement, unlike a fracture of the scaphoid where tenderness and swelling may often be minimal. In median nerve compression there is numbness of the thumb and the radial three to three and a half fingers, together with weakness or paralysis of the thenar muscles and the lateral two lumbricals.

Lateral x-ray shows the lunate either displaced forwards with the wrist intact, or the lunate in place and the whole wrist displaced backwards. In either case half the scaphoid, together with the lunate, may appear anterior to the other carpal bones.

On AP x-ray a dislocated lunate will appear **triangular** rather than its usual quadrilateral shape. If in doubt the opposite wrist should be x-rayed.

Reduction is achieved by prolonged traction followed by dorsiflexion of the wrist to open up the carpus. Pressure is then applied by the thumb on the dislocated lunate, and the wrist is flexed fully.

DISLOCATION OF THE LUNATE

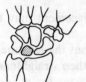

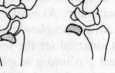

Normal Wrist
Quadrilateral Lunate

Dislocated Lunate
Triangular Lunate

REDUCTION

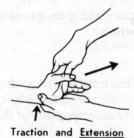

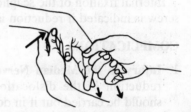

Traction and _Extension_ of Wrist
Pressure Over Lunate

Then

Flexion of Wrist with Traction and Pressure Over Lunate

OPEN OPERATION IF UNSUCCESSFUL

INITIAL IMMOBILISATION

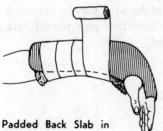

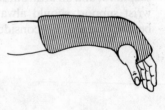

Padded Back Slab in Flexion for 3 Days Elevation

Complete Colles' Plaster in Flexion

The wrist is held flexed for 3 weeks with a back slab followed by a complete Colles type plaster. It is then held in a neutral position for a further 3 weeks.

If reduction fails, open operation and replacement may be necessary. Avascular changes may follow this.

In transcaphoid perilunar fracture dislocations the treatment is identical for the first 3 weeks. The wrist is then straightened and put into a scaphoid type skelecast or plaster for at least another 5 weeks, with full radial deviation. An above-elbow extension on the skelecast, with a hinge to limit the last 30 degress of extension, is helpful as this prevents rotation of the forearm.

Internal fixation of the scaphoid fracture with a compression screw is indicated if reduction is not perfect.

COMPLICATIONS

1. **Injury to the Median Nerve** — This usually settles after reduction of the dislocation. Electromyographic studies should be carried out if in doubt, and decompression of the nerve may be required.
2. **Avascular Necrosis of the Lunate** — Excision of the Lunate may be necessary, together with the proximal row of carpal bones, or prosthetic replacement of the lunate.
3. **Pain and Stiffness and Osteoarthritis** — Osteoarthritis may occur with avascular necrosis of the lunate or half the scaphoid, and an arthrodesis of the wrist may be indicated. A wrist support should always be tried, plus physiotherapy, before operation is considered.

DISLOCATION OF THE LUNATE

FURTHER TREATMENT
AFTER 3 WEEKS

Lunate Alone	Lunate + Scaphoid

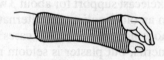

Colles Plaster with Wrist Straight for 3 Further Weeks	**Scaphoid Plaster or Skelecast** for **AT LEAST** **5 Further Weeks** Screw Scaphoid If Necessary

---

COMPLICATIONS

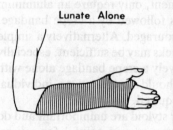

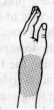
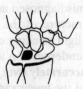

Wasting Thenar Median Nerve Compression	Incomplete Reduction	Stiff Painful Wrist	Avascular Necrosis Osteoarthritis
(S)	(S)	(P)	(S)

ISOLATED FRACTURES OF THE LOWER END OF THE RADIUS AND ULNA

Undisplaced fractures of the lower radius, or an impacted fracture with minimal displacement, only require an aluminum cock-up splint for 1 to 2 weeks followed by a crepe bandage. Early movements should be encouraged. Alternatively a simple skelecast support for about 3 weeks may be sufficient, especially in an older patient, or alternatively a crepe bandage alone with no other splinting. All cases should be treated on individual merits, but plaster is seldom required.

Isolated fractures of the ulnar styloid are unimportant and do not require treatment. They may remain painful for several weeks, and the patient should be warned about this. A detachable aluminium splint or crepe bandage alone may be necessary.

DE QUERVAIN'S SYNDROME

This is a painful tenosynovitis of the tendons of the abductor pollicis longus and extensor brevis tendons in their sheath over the lower end of the radius. This causes irritation and constriction in the tendon sheath with thickening of the tendon. This condition is often precipitated by trauma and may be misdiagnosed as a fracture of the lower end of the radius or as a fracture of the scaphoid itself. On examination there may be slight swelling over the lower end of the radial styloid. There is tenderness on abducting the thumb against resistance localised **accurately** over the radial styloid. X-ray may show osteoporosis of the lower radius in long-standing cases. Treatment is initially by injection with local anaesthetic and hydrocortisone. In over 50% this fails and decompression of the tendon sheaths may be necessary.

ISOLATED FRACTURES OF LOWER END OF RADIUS and ULNA

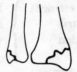

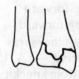

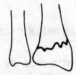

Usually Minimal or No Displacement
May Involve Joint

TREATMENT

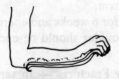

Usually does **NOT** Require Reduction
Treat with Aluminium Splint or
Crepe Bandage Alone for 3 weeks

COLLES FRACTURE OF THE WRIST

The "dinner fork" deformity in this fracture of the lower radius is caused by a fall on the outstretched hand.

1. **Backward** **displacement**	Lower Radius with	Impaction of the radius
2. **Backward** **rotation**		Fractures ulnar styloid (unimportant)
3. **Radial** **displacement**		Occasional other arm fractures

Reduction — This is achieved by **disimpacting well** by **prolonged** traction and then:

1. Pushing forward
2. Rotating forward   } Do **not** be afraid of over-reducing
3. Pushing ulna-wards

Hold Reduced — A 15cm back slab trimmed as illustrated, extending from knuckles to upper forearm. This should be in full pronation of the forearm, ulnar deviation of the wrist and neutral flexion. (Do **not** palmar flex, except in **difficult** fractures.)

Post Reduction —

1) The arm should be **well elevated** in a sling for a few days and the patient encouraged to move the fingers.
2) As soon as the swelling has subsided, (about 3 days) the plaster should be completed and the patient encouraged to use the hand and arm.
3) Immobilisation is for 6 weeks and energetic active exercises of the arm and shoulder should be encouraged in order to avoid stiffness.

Difficult and Unstable Fractures — In **very unstable** fractures **only** in **young** patients, hold fracture in full pronation in an **above**-elbow plaster.

COLLES FRACTURE

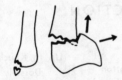

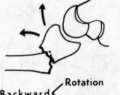

Lateral Displacement and
Impaction of Lower End
Radius,
Fracture Ulnar Styloid

Backward ⟨ Rotation
Displacement
Lower End Radius

REDUCTION

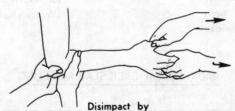

Disimpact by
Firm Traction under General Anaesthetic

Then

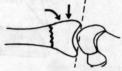

Push Ulnarwards
Pronate Wrist

Push Anteriorly
Rotate Anteriorly

Lower End of Radius
Normally Angled 10° Anteriorly

COLLES FRACTURE

POST-REDUCTION

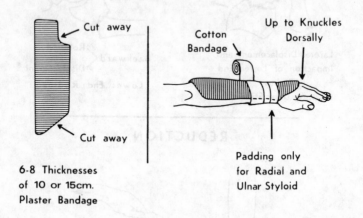

Cut away

Cut away

6-8 Thicknesses
of 10 or 15cm.
Plaster Bandage

Cotton
Bandage

Up to Knuckles
Dorsally

Padding only
for Radial and
Ulnar Styloid

RADIO-DORSAL BACK SLAB AND SLING

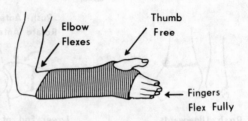

Elbow
Flexes

Thumb
Free

Fingers
Flex Fully

Complete Plaster when Swelling
has Subsided (3 Days +)

SLIPPED RADIAL EPIPHYSIS IN CHILDREN

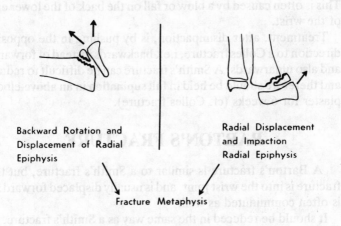

Backward Rotation and
Displacement of Radial
Epiphysis

Radial Displacement
and Impaction
Radial Epiphysis

Fracture Metaphysis

TREATMENT

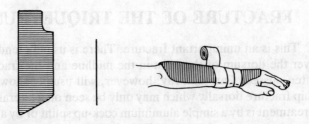

Reduce and Immobilise as for Colles Fracture

Plaster for 3-4 Weeks

Occasionally Kirschner Wire Fixation is Necessary

SMITH'S FRACTURE OF WRIST

A Smith's fracture is a reversed Colles fracture and the lower end of the radius is displaced forwards instead of backwards. This is often caused by a blow or fall on the back of the lower end of the wrist.

Treatment, after disimpaction, is by pushing in the opposite direction to a Colles fracture, i.e., backwards instead of forwards and also ulnarwards. A Smith's fracture can be difficult to reduce and therefore should be held in full **supination** in an **above**-elbow plaster for 6 weeks (cf. Colles fracture).

BARTON'S FRACTURE

A Barton's fracture is similar to a Smith's fracture, but the fracture is into the wrist joint, and is usually displaced forward. It is often comminuted as well.

It should be reduced in the same way as a Smith's fracture. In patients where a congruous joint cannot be achieved operative fixation may be required with a special T plate or occasionally Kirschner wires.

FRACTURE OF THE TRIQUETRUM

This is an unimportant fracture. There is usually tenderness over the dorsum of the wrist in the midline and the fracture is often missed. Careful x-ray, however, will usually show a tiny chip fracture dorsally which may only be seen on a lateral x-ray. Treatment is by a simple aluminium cock-up splint or by a Colles type skelecast for 3 weeks. **Minor** fractures of the other carpal bones are treated similarly.

SMITH'S FRACTURE
(REVERSED COLLES FRACTURE)

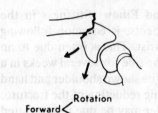

Rotation Forward
Displacement

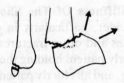

Lateral Displacement
and Impaction

REDUCTION

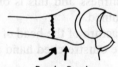

Push Back
Rotate Back

After Disimpacting SUPINATE Fully

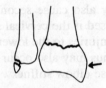

Push Ulnarwards

POST-REDUCTION

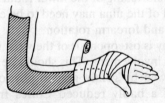

ABOVE Elbow Back Slab in **FULL SUPINATION**
Complete when Swelling has Subsided
Remove after **6 Weeks**
Watch for any Displacement of Fracture

COMPLICATIONS OF WRIST FRACTURES

Stiffness Of The Shoulder And Elbow: Stiffness in the shoulder, particularly in older patients, is common following Colles and other fractures of the wrist. This is often due to an elderly patient holding the arm to the side for several weeks in a sling, and all elderly patients should be shown shoulder and hand exercises to start on the day following reduction of the fracture. Occasionally stiffness of the shoulder may be due to associated injury to the shoulder or neck at the time of the fall on the outstretched hands. The shoulder and neck should, therefore, be examined in all cases of injury to the wrist. Cervical spondylosis may also cause secondary shoulder stiffness and this is often missed if the cervical spine is not examined.

Injuries to the lower humerus and fracture of the head of the radius may also occur with a fall on the outstretched hand and cause elbow stiffness.

Hand And Wrist Complications: Stiffness of the fingers is particularly common in old patients. This is due to lack of exercise plus immobilisation of the wrist **in flexion** in a Colles fracture.

Mal-union and shortening of the lower radius may also occur and the lower end of the ulna may need to be excised to regain both dorsiflexion and forearm rotation.

Sudeck's atrophy is osteoporosis of the wrist bones, probably due to autonomic involvement. This should be treated initially by rest and followed by gently graded physiotherapy. Other complications of a badly reduced Colles fracture include osteoarthritis, which may require physiotherapy, or occasionally a support or arthrodesis of the wrist. Rupture of the extensor pollicis longus tendon may occur and require tendon transfer of extensor indicis.

COMPLICATIONS OF FRACTURES OF LOWER END OF RADIUS and ULNA

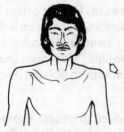

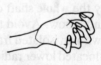

Stiffness of Fingers and Wrist Ⓟ

Stiffness of Shoulder due to Associated Injury or Prolonged Immobilisation Ⓟ

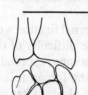

Sudeck's Atrophy

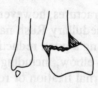

Malunion with Subluxation Radio-Ulnar Joint Excise Lower End Ulna Ⓢ

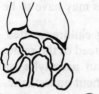

Osteoarthritis of Wrist Ⓟ

Wrist Support Arthrodesis Ⓢ

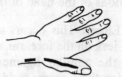

Rupture Extensor Pollicis Longus
↓
Transpose Extensor Indicis Ⓢ

FRACTURES OF THE SHAFT OF RADIUS AND ULNA

Diagnosis: This is usually straightforward. It is important always to x-ray the **whole** shaft of both radius and ulna to include **both** wrist and elbow. Avoid the trap of missing a dislocated head of radius with an isolated fracture of the ulna (Monteggia fracture), or a dislocated lower radio-ulnar joint with an isolated fracture of the radius (Galeazzi fracture).

Treatment: Traction and a well padded complete **above elbow** plaster, with the elbow at a right angle, should be tried. Fractures of the upper half usually require immobilisation in **supination,** and those of the lower half in **pronation** with elevation to prevent oedema.

Many fractures, however, require internal fixation with plates or intramedullary Rush nails due to the difficulty of obtaining and holding a good reduction. Physiotherapy, especially of the wrist and elbow, including rotation of the forearm, is essential after internal fixation or removal of the plaster after union has occurred.

Monteggia Fracture: This should be reduced and held in **forced** supination. Open reduction is often also necessary. Missed dislocations of the head of the radius may have to be excised.

Pulled Elbow: This occurs in young children, often due to a sudden jerk on the forearm, and the head of the radius subluxes out of the annular ligament. It can usually be reduced by supinating the forearm suddenly **without** anaesthetic.

FRACTURES OF THE SHAFT OF RADIUS and ULNA

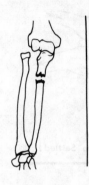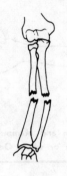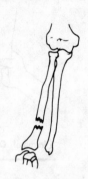

Fractured Ulna with Dislocation of Head of Radius (MONTEGGIA FRACTURE)

Fractured Radius and Ulnar Shaft

Fractured Radius with Dislocation of Lower Radio–Ulna Joint (GALEAZZI FRACTURE)

EMERGENCY TREATMENT

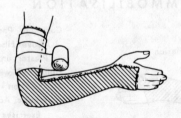

PADDED BACKSLAB and ELEVATION BEFORE MANIPULATION

FRACTURES OF THE SHAFT OF RADIUS and ULNA

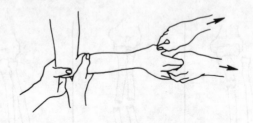

Traction and Manipulation
(Minimal Oedema or when Oedema Settled)

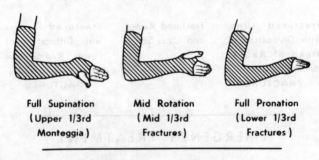

Full Supination
(Upper 1/3rd
Monteggia)

Mid Rotation
(Mid 1/3rd
Fractures)

Full Pronation
(Lower 1/3rd
Fractures)

IMMOBILISATION

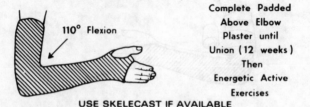

110° Flexion

Complete Padded
Above Elbow
Plaster until
Union (12 weeks)
Then
Energetic Active
Exercises

USE SKELECAST IF AVAILABLE

FRACTURES OF THE SHAFT OF RADIUS and ULNA

OPEN REDUCTION

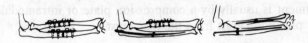

Plating Both
Radius and Ulna

Plate Radius
Intramedullary
Nail Ulna

Nail Both
Radius and Ulna

MONTEGGIA FRACTURE

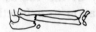

Excise

Fractured Ulna
with Dislocation of
Head of Radius

Plate or Nail Ulna
Reduce Head of
Radius

Nail or Plate Ulna
Excise Head of
Radius
(NOT IN CHILDREN)

GALEAZZI FRACTURE

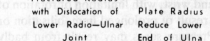
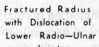

Excise

Fractured Radius
with Dislocation of
Lower Radio—Ulnar
Joint

Plate Radius
Reduce Lower
End of Ulna

OR

Plate Radius
Excise Lower
End of Ulna

COMPLICATIONS OF FRACTURES OF THE RADIUS AND ULNA

Non-Union: Non-union is particularly common in the lower third of the ulna where the blood supply is poor. It may also occur where the bone ends are not in contact, due to a rotation deformity or where the bone ends are being held apart. The treatment is usually by a compression plate or intramedullary nail, plus bone graft from the iliac crest.

MAL-UNION

Mal-union is particularly important, especially if more than 10 degrees angulation, as this will limit supination and pronation of the forearm. Internal fixation is necessary if a good position cannot be obtained by manipulation.

In cases where union has already occurred the degree of disability will determine whether any further treatment is justified. In cross union an osteotomy of the radius may occasionally be necessary to restore rotation to a functional position.

MISSED MONTEGGIA AND GALEAZZI FRACTURES

In isolated fractures of the upper ulna or lower radius dislocation of the head of the radius at the elbow or the lower end of the ulna at the wrist, respectively, can cause real disability in elbow or wrist movement. Excision of the head of the radius or the lower end of the ulna may be necessary, depending on the fracture.

OTHER COMPLICATIONS

Stiffness of the elbow and wrist, with limitation of rotation of the forearm, may be the result of prolonged immobilisation or lack of physiotherapy. Pressure sores may result from badly applied plasters.

FRACTURES OF THE SHAFT OF RADIUS and ULNA

COMPLICATIONS

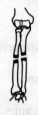

NON—UNION

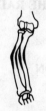

MAL—UNION

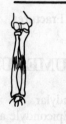

CROSS-UNION

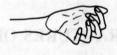

Complications due to
Too Tight Plaster, Plaster Sores
Volkmann's Ischaemic Contracture

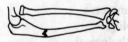

Untreated or Missed
Monteggia Fracture

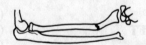

Untreated or Missed
Dislocated Lower
Radio—Ulnar Joint

Stiffness of Elbow and Wrist
Limitation of Rotation
of Forearm

DUE TO
{
Untreated Complications
Prolonged Immobilisation
Lack of Physiotherapy
}

INJURIES AROUND THE ELBOW
CLASSIFICATION

HEAD OF THE RADIUS
(1) Marginal Crack
(2) Comminution
(3) Dislocation

OLECRANON
(1) Minimal Displacement
(2) Separation
(3) Comminution

DISLOCATION OF ELBOW
(1) Without Fracture
(2) With Fracture of Coronoid process
(3) Multiple Fractures

FRACTURES OF THE HUMERUS

LOWER END
(1) Supracondylar
(2) Medial Epicondyle and Condyle
(3) Comminuted

SHAFT
(1) Transverse
(2) Oblique
(3) Pathological

UPPER END
(1) Fracture of Tuberosity
(2) Impacted Fracture of Neck
(3) Unimpacted Fracture of Neck
(4) Fracture plus Dislocation

FRACTURES OF THE HEAD OF RADIUS

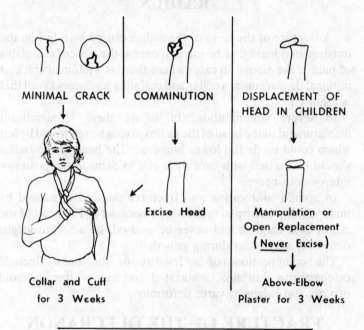

MINIMAL CRACK	COMMINUTION	DISPLACEMENT OF HEAD IN CHILDREN

Collar and Cuff for 3 Weeks	Excise Head	Manipulation or Open Replacement (Never Excise)

Above-Elbow Plaster for 3 Weeks

COMPLICATIONS

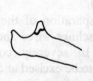

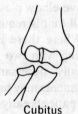

Osteoarthritis and Joint Stiffness	Associated Fracture of Coronoid Process	Cubitus Valgus

FRACTURE OF THE HEAD OF THE RADIUS

A fracture of the head of the radius caused by a fall on the outstretched hand may be missed, even if the patient complains of pain in the elbow. In cases where there is a minimal crack or minimal displacement a collar and cuff sling for 3 weeks is all that is required.

In severe comminution, or where there is significant displacement of the head of the radius, a rough area would be left which could erode the lower humerus. The head of the radius should be excised with care so as not to damage the posterior interosseous nerve.

In a child, dislocation and fractures should be reduced by manipulation and open reduction, if necessary. The head of the radius in a child should **never** be excised, or a severe valgus deformity may occur during growth.

The complications of a fracture of the radius include osteoarthritis, stiffness, associated fracture of the coronoid process and valgus or varus deformity.

FRACTURE OF THE OLECRANON

Fractures of the olecranon are usually due to a fall on the point of the elbow. In cases where there is no displacement an above-elbow plaster, or preferably skelecast, for about 6 weeks is all that is required.

Where there is separation of the olecranon, tension band wiring with two Kirschner wires and a figure-of-eight wire is usually necessary. In severely comminuted fractures the fragments may have to be excised and the triceps reattached. In old patients early movement without operation may occasionally be indicated.

The complications are illustrated and include severe osteoarthritis, joint stiffness, weakness of extension after excision of the olecranon, and established non-union.

FRACTURE OF THE OLECRANON

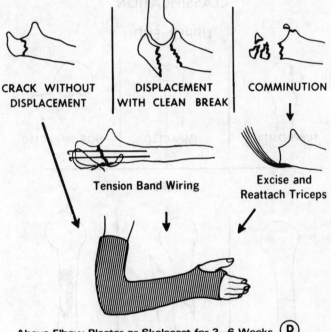

CRACK WITHOUT DISPLACEMENT

DISPLACEMENT WITH CLEAN BREAK

COMMINUTION

Tension Band Wiring

Excise and Reattach Triceps

Above Elbow Plaster or Skelecast for 3—6 Weeks (P)
ONLY IF FIXATION NOT STABLE

COMPLICATIONS

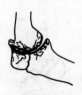

Osteoarthritis and Joint Stiffness

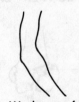

Weakness of Extension

Non—Union

FRACTURES OF THE HUMERUS
CLASSIFICATION

UPPER END

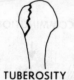

TUBEROSITY

IMPACTED

NOT IMPACTED

SHAFT

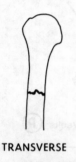

TRANSVERSE

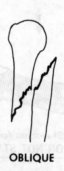

OBLIQUE

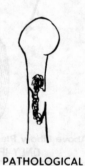

PATHOLOGICAL

LOWER END

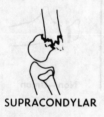

SUPRACONDYLAR

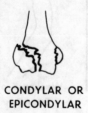

CONDYLAR OR EPICONDYLAR

COMMINUTED

FRACTURES OF THE HUMERUS
FIRST AID TREATMENT

UPPER and LOWER END	SHAFT	TRAVELLING A DISTANCE
	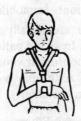	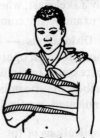
Sling	Collar and Cuff	Arm Bandaged to Side

ACUTE COMPLICATIONS

NECK and UPPER 1/3rd FRACTURES	MID 1/3 FRACTURES	LOWER 1/3rd FRACTURES
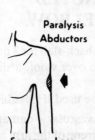	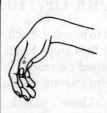	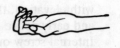

NECK and UPPER 1/3rd FRACTURES

Paralysis Abductors

Sensory Loss
Insertion Deltoid

Circumflex
Nerve Palsy

MID 1/3 FRACTURES

Wrist Drop

Radial
Nerve Palsy

LOWER 1/3rd FRACTURES

Vascular
Compression
Volkmann's
Ischaemic
Contracture
Gangrene

DISLOCATION OF ELBOW

Recent Dislocations — Reduce by traction or open reduction if this fails. Hold reduced with elbow at less than a right angle if possible. Use a well padded back-slab and complete this, or apply a skelecast, when the swelling has settled. Watch the pulse and examine for complications. Immobilise for 3 weeks.

Old Dislocations — These are usually impossible to reduce without an open operation. In an old patient, no operation may be necessary. In manual labourers or young men, arthrodesis of the elbow may be indicated. Arthroplasty of the elbow joint may be indicated, particularly in the elderly.

Complications of the Dislocated Elbow -

(1) **Traumatic Ossification** — This should be treated by further immobilisation.
(2) **Associated Fractures** — These should be treated.
(3) **Vascular and Nerve Damage** — See supracondylar fracture.

SEVERELY COMMINUTED FRACTURE OF THE ELBOW

Treatment — Admit to hospital. Padded back-slab for 3 days with elevation, then firm crepe bandage over wool, a sling and early active assisted exercises.
Internal screw or wire fixation should be used if possible.

Complications — These include vascular damage, Volkmann's ischaemic contracture, gangrene of the arm and neurological damage, especially of the ulnar nerve. Osteoarthritis, stiffness and deformity may occur, as described, with condylar fractures.

LOWER END OF HUMERUS
LATERAL CONDYLE

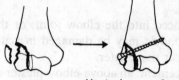

COMPLICATIONS

Cubitus Valgus
Late Ulnar Nerve Palsy
Osteoarthritis

Manipulate or **Screw**
Above Elbow Plaster
for 6 Weeks

COMMINUTED FRACTURES

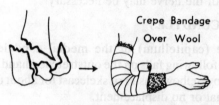

Crepe Bandage
Over Wool

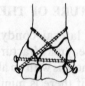

Olecranon Traction   or (S) Internally Fix
(Kirschner Wire)   if Possible

DISLOCATED ELBOW

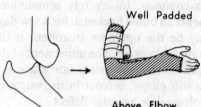

Well Padded

COMPLICATIONS

Associated Fractures
Vascular and
Neurological Damage
**Traumatic
Ossification**

Above Elbow
Plaster or
Back Slab

FRACTURE OF THE CONDYLES OF THE HUMERUS

MEDIAL EPICONDYLE

The condyle may be displaced into the elbow joint, or the ulnar nerve behind the epicondyle may be damaged in acute fractures, or constricted by scar tissue later.

If there is little or no displacement, an above-elbow plaster or skelecast should be used. In severe displacement manipulation should be attempted. If unsuccessful, open operation and resuturing in place, or Kirschner wire fixation, may be required.

Complications include damage to the ulnar nerve, and ulnar neuritis due to scarring and adhesions at the site of the fracture. Anterior transposition of the nerve may be necessary.

FRACTURE OF THE CONDYLES

The lateral condyle (capitellum) or the medial condyle (trochlea) may fracture following falls on the outstretched hand. Treatment is with an above-elbow plaster or skelecast for about 6 weeks if there is minimal or no displacement.

If displacement is of any significant degree the condyle should be reduced and held either with 2 or 3 Kirschner wires, or with one or more compression screws.

In comminuted fractures attempts should be made to screw all the fragments together, or hold them with Kirschner wires, otherwise osteoarthritis is common. In severely comminuted fractures with many fragments an initial back-slab for a few days and early movements may be the optimum treatment if the fragments are too comminuted to replace. The movement of the elbow will mould the fragments to some extent into place.

Complications include a stiff elbow, osteoarthritis, valgus or varus deformity and neurological or vascular defect.

FRACTURE OF THE EPICONDYLE

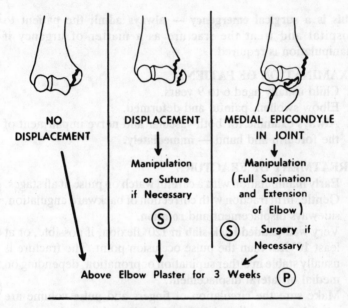

NO DISPLACEMENT	DISPLACEMENT	MEDIAL EPICONDYLE IN JOINT
	Manipulation or Suture if Necessary ⓢ	Manipulation (Full Supination and Extension of Elbow) Surgery if Necessary ⓢ

Above Elbow Plaster for 3 Weeks Ⓟ

COMPLICATIONS

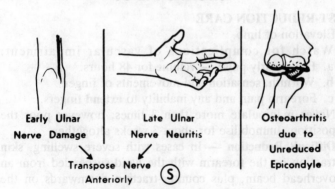

Early Ulnar Nerve Damage	Late Ulnar Nerve Neuritis	Osteoarthritis due to Unreduced Epicondyle
	Transpose Nerve Anteriorly ⓢ	

SUPRACONDYLAR FRACTURE OF HUMERUS

This is a surgical emergency — always admit the patient to hospital and treat the fracture as a matter of urgency if manipulation is required.

EXAMINATION OF PATIENT
1. Child usually aged 6 to 9 years.
2. Elbow swollen, painful and deformed.
3. Always examine for both vascular and nerve impairment of the forearm and hand — **immediately.**

TREATMENT OF FRACTURE
1. Early manipulation with a careful watch on pulse at all stages. Gentle, firm traction with correction of backward angulation, sideways displacement and **rotation.**
2. Very **well-padded back-slab** in 120° flexion, if possible, or at least 10° **less** than the pulse occlusion point. The fracture is usually stable in either supination or pronation, depending on medial or lateral displacement.
3. Make sure the circulation of fingers and **pulse** volume are good **before** sending the patient back to the ward.

POST-REDUCTION CARE
1. Elevation of limb.
2. Watch for complications of vascular impairment:
   a. Half-hourly pulse — **volume** for 48 hours.
   b. Warmth, sensation and movements of fingers.
   c. Forearm pain and any inability to **extend** fingers.
3. Never manipulate more than 3 times, however poor the position. Immobilise for about 3 weeks altogether.
4. **Difficult Reduction** — In cases with severe swelling, skin traction on the forearm with the hand suspended from an overhead beam, plus counter-traction downwards on the upper arm with a sling for about 3 days.
   (See illustration). Occasionally immobilise in extension.

SUPRACONDYLAR FRACTURE

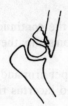 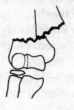

REDUCTION

Careful Observation of Radial Pulse	Admit to Hospital	Lateral or Medial Displacement Corrected
Supination or Pronation for Stability		
Traction		Immobilisation in Extension (Special Cases) ONLY

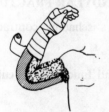

POST REDUCTION

Elbow 110°
If Possible
PULSE MUST
BE GOOD

Well Padded
Split Plaster
Observation
in Hospital

1/2 hourly Check ⎤ Warmth Sensation
Fingers ⎬ Ability to Extend
Pulse Volume ⎦ with Minimal Pain
DIFFICULT CASES - SKIN TRACTION

VASCULAR IMPAIRMENT

1. **Immediately** remove plaster and extend the elbow.
2. **Prepare theatre.**
3. **Operate immediately unless** sure of the **continued return** of the circulation. Do **NOT** waste time on sympathetic blocks or vasodilators.

Exposure — Incise lower third of upper arm and most of the forearm over artery. Split fascia and lacertus fibrosus. **NO** tourniquet.

Brachial Artery — Identify artery medial to biceps tendon and bathe with warm 2.5% papaverine or 50 mg of pethidine in 10ml of warm saline. If the artery is severely lacerated or divided try to suture the two ends. If impossible, consider inserting a vein graft in the reverse direction. If the artery remains constricted and pale, the lumen should **always** be exposed. Intimal damage is common in these cases and may not be apparent on external exposure of the artery. Resection and anastomosis or grafting may be necessary.

Closure of Wound — Close **skin** only and **only** if this can be done easily. Otherwise leave centre of wound open and perform a secondary suture in about 3 days.

COMPLICATIONS OF SUPRACONDYLAR FRACTURE

1. **Vascular Impairment** — Volkmann's ischaemic contracture or gangrene of arm.
2. **Traumatic Ossification.**
3. **Cubitus varus** (poor appearance and function), or **cubitus valgus** (late ulnar palsy).

SUPRACONDYLAR FRACTURE

EARLY COMPLICATIONS

TREATMENT OF ISCHAEMIA OF FOREARM

No Tourniquet

Extend Elbow

Skin Incision

Split Deep Fascia in Forearm Carefully for Whole length

OR

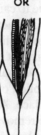

Biceps Tendon Guide to Artery

Split Lacertus Fibrosus

Bathe Artery in Spasm with 2·5% Papaverine or Pethidine

OPEN ARTERY IN MOST CASES

EMERGENCY - REMOVE PLASTER AND OPERATE WITHIN 1 HOUR

Lacerated Artery

Ligate or Graft or End to End Suture

Further Treatment

Never Suture Fascia Delayed Primary Suture Skin Reduce Fracture

LATE COMPLICATIONS

CUBITUS VARUS OR VALGUS

TRAUMATIC OSSIFICATION OR STIFFNESS

FRACTURES OF THE SHAFT OF HUMERUS

Fractures of the shaft of the humerus may be caused by a fall on the outstretched hand, or they may be due to direct trauma. Secondary deposits due to carcinoma also commonly involve the shaft of the humerus. In fractures of the shaft, a collar and cuff sling and **not** a triangular sling is required. This will allow the weight of the arm to distract the fragments and allow alignment, as the effect of gravity will pull against the muscles. In addition a simple plaster slab applied over wool will support the arm and this is bandaged into place. As soon as the swelling has subsided the bandage should be removed and a complete plaster applied.

Alternatively a slab alone for 3 or 4 weeks, followed by a tight fitting lightweight plastic splint, is a more comfortable alternative for the patient, and the fracture usually takes from 8 to 12 weeks to unite. In very unstable fractures the arm should be held in an abduction splint in 60° abduction. In cases with gross displacement, internal fixation with a nail or plate may be required.

If there is a radial nerve palsy, this can be treated in most cases conservatively by a simple cock-up splint, and over 80% of cases will recover. A "lively" splint to keep the fingers extended is indicated where recovery does not occur in 2 or 3 weeks. Exploration of the radial nerve is indicated in cases where there is no recovery or where there is evidence of division or pressure by bone on the nerve.

In established non-union or difficult fractures, a simple shoulder abduction splint with the arm held with circular strips of fibreglass should be tried initially. If this is unsuccessful, internal fixation with a compression plate and bone grafting or a Huckstep or Rush nail may be required.

In pathological fractures due to secondary deposits from carcinoma a simple Rush nail should be inserted blind from the tuberosity, under image intensifier control, followed by deep X-ray therapy.

FRACTURE SHAFT HUMERUS

TREATMENT

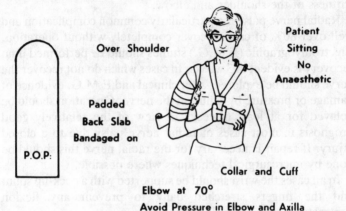

Patient
Sitting
No
Anaesthetic

Over Shoulder

P.O.P:

Padded
Back Slab
Bandaged on

Collar and Cuff
Elbow at 70°
Avoid Pressure in Elbow and Axilla

FURTHER TREATMENT

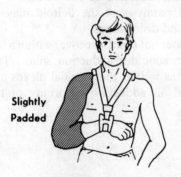

Slightly
Padded

8-12 Weeks
Average
Physiotherapy
to Mobilise
Shoulder
and Elbow

Complete Plaster
When Oedema
Settled

COMPLICATIONS

The main complications are damage to the circumflex and radial nerves and non-union. Other complications include stiffness of the shoulder and elbow.

Radial nerve palsy is a particularly common complication and well over 80% of cases recover completely without operation. Electromyographic (E.M.G.) studies should be performed if no recovery is evident in 3 weeks. In cases which do not recover the nerve should be explored, after clinical and E.M.G. evidence of damage or pressure by callus on the nerve. Operation should be delayed for at least 6 weeks in view of the relatively good prognosis in most cases of radial nerve palsy due to a closed injury. If repair is necessary for the radial nerve this should be done by microsurgical techniques where possible.

In all cases the wrist should be supported with a cock-up splint and the fingers stretched daily to prevent any flexion contractures with a "lively" splint.

Circumflex nerve palsy may occur with fractures of the upper end of the humerus and with dislocation of the shoulder. Diminished sensation over the **insertion** of the deltoid is an indication of this, as actual paralysis of the deltoid may be difficult to test in fractures and dislocations.

A circumflex palsy which does not rapidly recover within a few days should be treated in a shoulder abduction splint. This relaxes the circumflex nerve as well as the brachial plexus and diminishes the likelihood of an adduction deformity of the shoulder.

FRACTURE SHAFT HUMERUS COMPLICATIONS

MUSCLE INTERPOSITION and DELAYED UNION

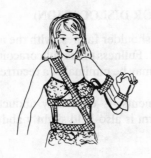

Skelecast Abduction Splint

Manipulation under Anaesthetic if Necessary

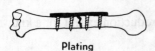 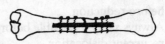

Plating

Huckstep Intramedullary Nail

RADIAL NERVE PALSY | CIRCUMFLEX PALSY

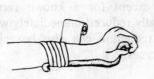 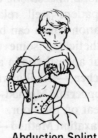

Cock - Up Splint and Daily Stretching

Abduction Splint

DISLOCATION OF SHOULDER

CLASSIFICATION

1. Anterior — Subcoracoid.
2. Inferior — Luxatio Erecta — rare.
3. Posterior — Post Glenoid — uncommon.

EXAMINATION (ANTERIOR DISLOCATION)

1. Flattening of the normal shoulder fullness with the acromion the most prominent point. Fullness in the subcoracoid region.
2. Pain and swelling — this may be minimal in a recurrent or old dislocation.
3. Limitation of all movements — especially abduction and external rotation. The arm is also held slightly abducted.

INVESTIGATION

1. Always look for complications, i.e., circumflex nerve palsy, associated fracture, brachial plexus injury or vascular damage **before** reduction.
2. Always x-ray if possible before reduction except for a known **recurrent** dislocation.

REDUCTION (See Illustrations)

General anaesthetic or Valium and Pethidine intravenously, with patient well relaxed, except for a known **recurrent** dislocation which can be usually reduced immediately without anaesthetic. In some cases reduction can also be achieved without anaesthetic in acute cases.

1. **Kocher** — As illustrated.
2. **Hippocratic Method** — The **un**booted (!) foot in the axilla and a seat on the floor.
3. **Relaxation Method** — Patient lying face down on couch with arm hanging down. This may sometimes spontaneously reduce a dislocation with minimal assistance.

DISLOCATED SHOULDER

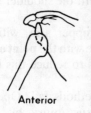

Anterior

Fracture Dislocation

Posterior

EXAMINATION
(Anterior Dislocation)

Arm Abducted

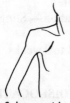

Subcoracoid Fullness Anteriorly

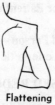

Flattening Posteriorly

ACUTE COMPLICATIONS

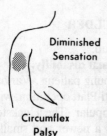

Diminished Sensation

Circumflex Palsy

Nerve or Arterial Damage

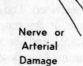

Neck or Tuberosity

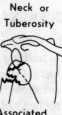

Associated Fracture

4. **Other Methods**
   a. Very good relaxant anaesthesia and lift the shoulder back into its socket.
   b. A padded broad sling around the upper arm, with an assistant pulling laterally and pressure with the **point of the elbow** over the head of the humerus to reduce this back into the glenoid.
   c. Open reduction when the above methods fail. Operate rather than cause a brachial plexus injury by over enthusiastic manipulation.

POST-REDUCTION

1. **Young Person** — Wool pad in axilla and arm to the side for 3 weeks in collar and cuff method as illustrated.
2. **Old Person or Patient with Recurrent Dislocation** — Sling for 3 days.
3. **Middle Aged Person** — Arm to the side for 1 to 3 weeks. Then in all cases, energetic active exercises.

FAILED CLOSED REDUCTION AND OLD DISLOCATION

1. **Young Patient** — with recent dislocation — open reduction.
2. **Old Patient** — with marked stiffness — open reduction.
3. **Old Unreduced Dislocation** — consider doing nothing except give shoulder exercises. Arthrodesis may be indicated, or possibly a prosthesis.

RECURRENT DISLOCATION OF SHOULDER

The following treatment is recommended.
1. **Do nothing in an old person with minimal disability.**
2. **Operate** if more than 3 dislocations in young patients. Various operations have been described. The Putti-Platt operation, with "reefing" of the capsule, is the most popular. The Huckstep single hole titanium staple and screw is a newer and smaller operation and allows immediate post-operative movements.

DISLOCATED SHOULDER TREATMENT

AFTER X-RAY

KOCHER MANOEUVRE

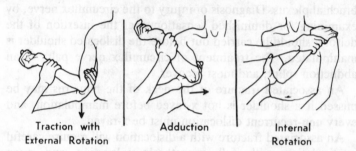

| Traction with External Rotation | Adduction | Internal Rotation |

HIPPOCRATIC METHOD

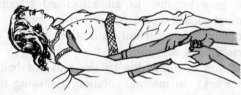

Gentle Traction
Adduction over
Unbooted Foot

Patient on Ground

Open Reduction if Above Methods Fail

POST REDUCTION

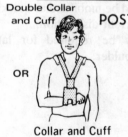

Double Collar and Cuff

OR

Collar and Cuff

3 Weeks — Young Patient

3 Days — Old Patient and Recurrent Dislocation

then

Energetic Physiotherapy

COMPLICATIONS OF DISLOCATED SHOULDER

Early complications include injury to the circumflex nerve, associated fracture of the neck of the humerus and injury to the brachial plexus. Diagnosis of injury to the circumflex nerve, by examining for diminished sensation over the insertion of the deltoid, should be carried out before the dislocated shoulder is manipulated. The treatment of circumflex nerve palsy is an abduction splint, and most recover.

An associated fracture of the neck of the humerus may be missed if a shoulder is not x-rayed before manipulation, and every **non**-recurrent dislocation must be x-rayed.

An associated fracture with a dislocation will require careful manipulation with full anaesthesia relaxation and open reduction plus internal fixation of the fracture if not successful. Injury to the brachial plexus usually follows too forceful a manipulation, but may be due to an associated fracture dislocation. Treatment should include an abduction splint.

Late complications include recurrent dislocation, stiffness of the shoulder and circumflex nerve injury.

Recurrent dislocation is often due to the arm not being immobilised for 3 weeks, in internal rotation, following the initial reduction in a younger patient.

Stiffness of the shoulder is common in old patients in whom the shoulder is immobilised for more than 1 to 2 weeks. In elderly patients, therefore, the shoulder should be mobilised as quickly as possible, even at the risk of a recurrent dislocation.

Arthrodesis of the shoulder may be required for late circumflex palsy or stiffness of the shoulder.

SHOULDER INJURIES
COMPLICATIONS

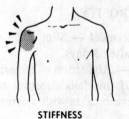

**STIFFNESS
AND PAIN**

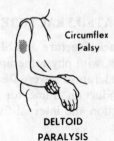

Circumflex
Palsy

**DELTOID
PARALYSIS**

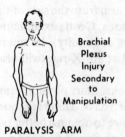

Brachial
Plexus
Injury
Secondary
to
Manipulation

PARALYSIS ARM

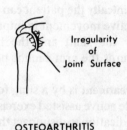

Irregularity
of
Joint Surface

OSTEOARTHRITIS

TREATMENT FOR RECURRENT DISLOCATION

HUCKSTEP STAPLE & SCREW

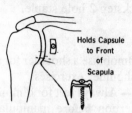

Holds Capsule
to Front
of
Scapula

**Immediate Movement
Permitted**

Putti-Platt Operation

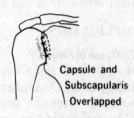

Capsule and
Subscapularis
Overlapped

FRACTURE OF UPPER END OF HUMERUS

ISOLATED FRACTURE OF TUBEROSITY

Crack Fracture and Slight Displacement — Sling for 1 to 2 weeks, with physiotherapy starting after 3 days.

Moderate or Severe Displacement — Abduction of the arm in an abduction frame for 3 weeks. If this fails consider open reduction and internal fixation in severe cases with a screw or staple.

FRACTURES OF NECK OF HUMERUS

Clinically the patient **can** lift the arm from the side of the body by active movement in impacted cases. **Gentle** examination may show the shaft and the head in continuity. In unimpacted fractures the arm cannot be lifted at all. X-rays will also be of help.

Treatment is by a sling for 3 weeks. Start physiotherapy with gentle active assisted exercises after 3 days. There is almost **never** an indication to disimpact the fracture to obtain a better position.

In unimpacted fractures in a young or middle aged patient, a manipulation under general anaesthesia with impaction of the two ends should be attempted, then a sling for 3 weeks. Occasionally immobilisation in a shoulder spica is necessary or fixation with a Rush nail or a Huckstep 2 hole staple.

COMPLICATIONS

1. **Stiffness of Shoulder** — **Never** immobilise a shoulder for more than 3 weeks and always give shoulder exercises.
2. **Injury to the Circumflex Nerve** — Always test for diminished sensation over the deltoid insertion **before** manipulation. Give early exercises and an abduction frame if necessary.
3. **Associated Dislocation of the Shoulder** — Gentle manipulation, but operative reduction may be necessary.

FRACTURE UPPER END HUMERUS

TREATMENT

TUBEROSITY WITH MINIMAL OR NO DISPLACEMENT	IMPACTED	DISPLACEMENT IN OLD PATIENT

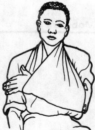

Triangular Sling
ONLY for
1 - 3 weeks
1 WEEK — Old Patients
3 Weeks -Young Patients

No Manipulation
Early Active
Assisted Shoulder
Exercises

FRACTURE SCAPULA

Triangular Sling for 1–3 Weeks	Early Active Assisted Shoulder Exercises	Rarely Requires Manipulation or Surgery

(P)

FRACTURE UPPER END HUMERUS

COMPLICATIONS

DISPLACEMENT
IN YOUNG PATIENT

↓

Manipulation and
Sling or Spica
Open Reduction
if Necessary

OLD PATIENT - Sling Mobilise

TUBEROSITY WITH
DISPLACEMENT

↓

Manipulation
and Spica
3 Weeks
Screw if Necessary

FRACTURE DISLOCATION

→

Gentle Manipulation
and Sling or Spica
3 Weeks

Open Reduction
if Necessary

CIRCUMFLEX PALSY

Area Diminished
Sensation Insertion
of Deltoid

→

Shoulder Exercises
+
Spica or
Abduction Splint
for
Deltoid Palsy

ROTATOR CUFF INJURIES

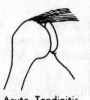

Acute Tendinitis | Partial Rupture | Complete Rupture

DIAGNOSIS

Inability to Initiate Abduction

Inject Local Anaesthetic

Partial Rupture
Can Now Lift Arm

Complete Rupture
Still No Abduction

X-ray for Calcification

TREATMENT

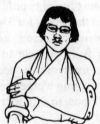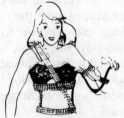

Sling + Physiotherapy
for Tendinitis or
Partial Rupture

Shoulder Spica
for Complete Rupture
+ Repair in Young Patient

INJURIES TO ACROMIO —
CLAVICULAR JOINT

These are caused by a fall on the point of the shoulder. **Always** examine the acromio-clavicular as well as the coraco-clavicular ligaments. If in doubt take an A.P. x-ray of **both** acromio-clavicular joints.

Sprain — Tenderness and slight swelling over the joint. No displacement. Treatment is by a triangular sling for 3 days and shoulder exercises.

Subluxation — The weak acromio-clavicular ligament is ruptured, but the strong conoid and trapezoid ligaments remain intact. There is tenderness and swelling over the joint and an increase in the normal "step" between the lateral end of the clavicle and the acromion, reduced easily by pressing up on the elbow. X-rays show subluxation of the acromio-clavicular joint, but no increase in the gap between coracoid and clavicle. Triangular sling for 1 to 3 weeks.

Dislocation — All 3 ligaments, acromio-clavicular, conoid and trapezoid are ruptured. There is some swelling and pain, and a large reducible step between clavicle and acromion with a gap between the coracoid and clavicle. Most patients only require a triangular sling supporting the point of the elbow for 3 weeks and shoulder exercises. A Kirschner wire or screw across the acromio-clavicular joint, or a screw from clavicle to coracoid process with fascial repair or reinforcement is occasionally indicated in athletes using this arm or young women requiring a "cosmetic" shoulder. Strapping from elbow to shoulder is **seldom** tolerated.

Complications — Few complications occur other than the cosmetic one. The outer end of the clavicle occasionally requires later excision for cosmesis.

ACROMIO-CLAVICULAR DISLOCATION

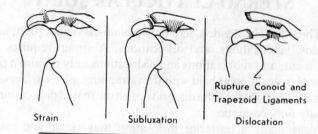

Strain

Subluxation

Dislocation
Rupture Conoid and
Trapezoid Ligaments

TREATMENT

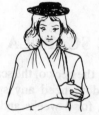

Sling Alone
Strain and Subluxation
Most Dislocations

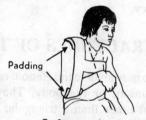

Padding

T. Support for 3 Weeks
(Dislocation Sometimes)
<u>Doubtful</u> Value

OTHER TREATMENT
(Dislocations - Young Patients)

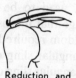

Reduction and
Kirschner Wire

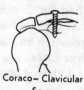

Coraco-Clavicular
Screw

Excision Outer End
Clavicle
Late Cases Only

MOST PATIENTS REQUIRE TRIANGULAR SLING <u>ALONE</u>

INJURIES OF THE STERNO-CLAVICULAR JOINT

These may be divided, like the acromio-clavicular joint, into sprains, subluxations, and dislocations. A sprain requires no treatment, and subluxations and dislocations only require a pad of wool over the joint held with firm strapping, plus a triangular sling for 1 to 3 weeks. The disability of an untreated dislocation is usually only cosmetic.

Occasionally a posterior dislocation may occur and cause pressure on the vessels at the base of the neck. It will require reduction and stabilization with Kirschner wires as a surgical emergency.

FRACTURES OF THE SCAPULA

These may involve the glenoid cavity, the neck of the scapula, the acromion, or the body. They seldom need any specific treatment other than a triangular sling for 3 weeks and early shoulder exercises.

FRACTURES OF THE CLAVICLE

These usually occur at the junction of the medial two-thirds and the lateral one-third. A **well-padded** figure-of-eight bandage, plus triangular sling for 3 weeks, used to be the standard treatment, but it has the disadvantage that it loosens and requires frequent reapplication and is seldom required.

The **best treatment,** in most cases, is a triangular sling **only** under the clothing for 3 days, followed by a triangular sling over the clothes for 2 or 3 weeks.

Complications include injury to the apex of the lung, and subclavian vein. Non-union may occur, but is uncommon. A lump due to callus only rarely necessitates operation.

STERNO - CLAVICULAR DISLOCATION

Strain

Subluxation

Dislocation

TREATMENT

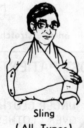

Sling
(All Types)

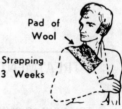

Pad of Wool

Strapping
3 Weeks

Local Pressure
(Subluxation and Dislocation)

OTHER TREATMENT
(Dislocation Only)

Reconstruction Sterno-Clavicular Ligament

Kirschner Wire

Open Reduction

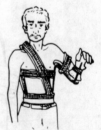

Abduction Splint

FRACTURES OF THE CLAVICLE

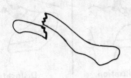

Commonly Junction
Inner 2/3rds Outer 1/3rd

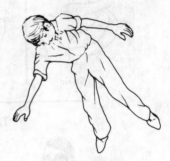

Fall on Outstretched Hand

TREATMENT IN MOST PATIENTS

TRIANGULAR SLING

UNDER CLOTHES 3 DAYS
OVER CLOTHES 3 WEEKS

MOST CASES

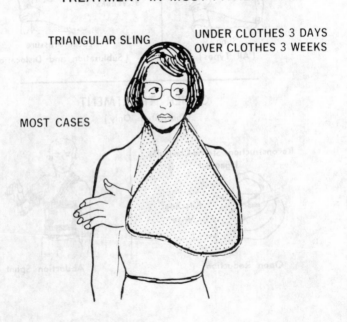

FRACTURES OF THE CLAVICLE

FIGURE OF EIGHT

FIGURE OF EIGHT

ONLY IN FEW CASES
WITH SEVERE OVERLAP

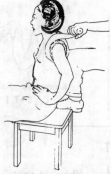

(DOUBTFUL VALUE)

Adequate Wool

Under Arms

NOT
TOO Wide

Shoulder Braced Well Back

COMPLICATIONS

**UNSIGHTLY
DEFORMITY**

NON-UNION

**SOFT TISSUE
INJURY**

Rare

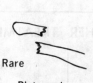

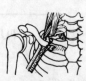

Rarely Require
Trimming

Plate and
Bone Graft (S)

Apex Lung Vessels
Nerves

BRACHIAL PLEXUS INJURIES
BIRTH INJURIES

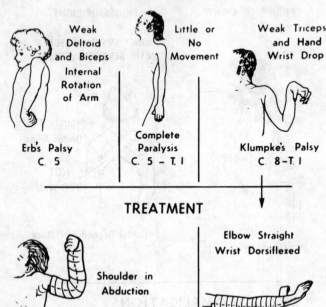

Weak Deltoid and Biceps Internal Rotation of Arm

Little or No Movement

Weak Triceps and Hand Wrist Drop

Erb's Palsy
C. 5

Complete Paralysis
C. 5 – T. 1

Klumpke's Palsy
C. 8 – T. 1

TREATMENT

Shoulder in Abduction

Elbow Straight Wrist Dorsiflexed

Above Elbow Back Slab

Above Elbow Slab

FURTHER TREATMENT

Daily Passive Stretching All Muscle Groups

Ⓟ

Reconstructive Surgery
↓
Late

Ⓢ

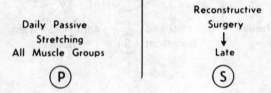

BRACHIAL PLEXUS INJURIES
CHILDREN AND ADULTS

CAUSES

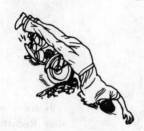

Fall on Point of Shoulder

Brachial Plexus
Torn –
Usually Complete
and
Preaxonal

DIAGNOSIS

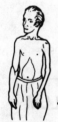

Flail or
Weak Arm

Changed
Electrical
Response

Absent or
Diminished
Sensation
and Sweating

Histamine Test
Positive Wheal and Flare
= Preaxonal Damage –
Poor Prognosis

Negative Test
= Postaxonal Damage–
Better Prognosis

E.M.G. in ALL CASES

TREATMENT

Exploration
and Repair
Only in some
Postaxonal Cases

Physiotherapy
Energetic and
Early Passive
Movements

Later
Reconstruction
Nerve Graft
or Amputation

DIFFICULT FRACTURES

SUPRACONDYLAR

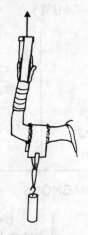

Before and
after Reduction

Extend Elbow as Necessary
Flex Elbow plus Plaster after 48 - 72 hours

TROCHLEA OR CAPITELLUM

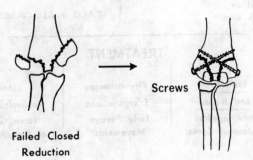

Screws

Failed Closed
Reduction

DIFFICULT FRACTURES

DISLOCATED LUNATE +
FRACTURE 1/2 SCAPHOID

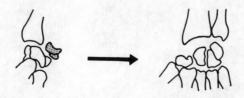

Failed Closed
Reduction

Excise Proximal
Row Carpal Bones

FRACTURE DISLOCATION
SHOULDER

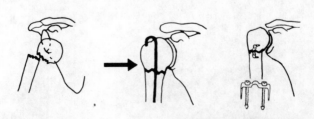

Failed Closed
Reduction

Open Reduction +
Intramedullary Nail

or

Huckstep Two Hole Staple

SPINE

FRACTURES OF THE SPINE

CAUSATION

ASSOCIATED WITH HEAD

FORCED FLEXION — FORCED EXTENSION, INJURY with or without Rotation

Dorsal Spine

COMPRESSION FRACTURE

FORCED FLEXION

FALL ON FEET - FALL FROM HEIGHT, ROTATION OF SPINE

ASSOCIATED INJURIES

DISLOCATED HIP AND PELVIS   CALCANEUS   HEAD INJURY

FRACTURES OF THE SPINE
CAUSATION

Entire Spine

Cervical Spine

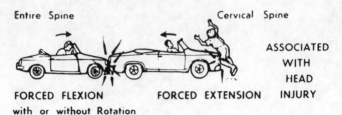

ASSOCIATED
WITH
HEAD
INJURY

FORCED FLEXION
with or without Rotation

FORCED EXTENSION

Entire Spine

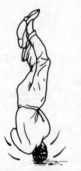

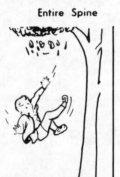

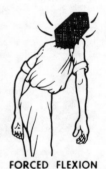

FALL ON HEAD

FALL FROM HEIGHT

FORCED FLEXION
ROTATION OF SPINE

ASSOCIATED INJURIES

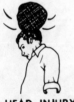

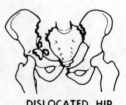

HEAD INJURY

CALCANEUS

DISLOCATED HIP
AND PELVIS

FRACTURES OF THE SPINE

CAUSATION

Fractures of the spine are often caused by a flexion plus rotation strain, particularly in the cervical and thoraco-lumbar regions.

In the cervical region many fractures are associated with head injuries and are frequently not diagnosed in unconscious patients. It is essential, in all head injuries, to treat the patient on suspicion. Forced flexion of the cervical spine, particularly associated with rotation, may cause a dislocation, a fracture dislocation or a fracture of one or both facets or the odontoid peg.

A hyperextension injury of the cervical spine, also called whiplash injury, is common in rear car collisions, particularly if the occupants of the car do not have high enough head restraints, or none at all.

Fractures and even dislocations in the cervical region due to the wide canal, may not necessarily be associated with cord damage, but root pressure is common.

Fractures of the thoracic spine are particularly common in flexion and flexion rotation injuries, and paralysis with complete cord transection is common due to the tight fit of the cord in the relatively small spinal canal.

Fractures of the thoraco-lumbar regions are common due to a flexion rotation strain and may cause both cord and root damage.

Fractures in the lumbar region may affect the conus or cauda equina and are commonly associated with falls from a height. They may be associated with fractures of the calcaneus. It is important to look for autonomic damage and particularly an inability to micturate following these injuries, and perineal numbness.

FRACTURES OF THE SPINE

INJURIES CERVICAL SPINE

EMERGENCY TRANSPORT

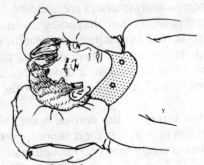

Watch for
Respiratory
Distress
Treat Other
Injuries

Head Flat on Stretcher
Sandbags on Each Side
of Head to Support Head

Cervical Collar if Available

PLASTAZOTE COLLAR IF AVAILABLE

EMERGENCY TREATMENT

GLISSON'S SLING

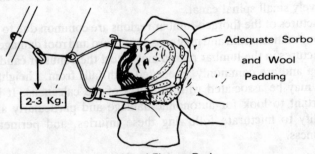

2-3 Kg.

Adequate Sorbo
and Wool
Padding

Head Flat on Bed
Mattress on Fracture Boards
Sandbags to Support Head

FRACTURES OF THE SPINE
EMERGENCY TRANSPORT
THORACIC AND LUMBAR SPINE

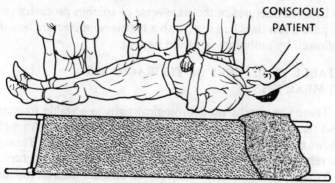

CONSCIOUS PATIENT

JORDAN FRAME

Lift Patient Flat on Back
Spinal Board if Available

UNCONSCIOUS PATIENT

Keep Airway

Clear

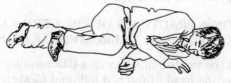

Elevate Foot of
Stretcher

[Only for
Short Periods]

Patient Flat On Face
Splint Other Injuries

SPINAL FRACTURES WITHOUT NEUROLOGICAL SIGNS

MINOR FRACTURES

Isolated fractures of the transverse or spinous processes only require a few days bed rest, with a mattress on fracture boards, followed by mobilisation of the patient.

STABLE FRACTURES OF THORACIC AND LUMBAR SPINES

There are usually no neurological signs in a stable fracture, and the supra and interspinous ligaments are intact. An x-ray shows **no** slipping forward of one vertebra on the next. There is merely compression of the vertebral body or a chip fracture.

Treatment should be by bed rest **flat** on a mattress on fracture boards for a few days. Back extension exercises should be given if possible.

The patient occasionally requires a back support such as a Taylor brace (this also supports the shoulder and chest) or a lumbo-sacral brace, for a variable period from 1 to 3 months, and perhaps longer, depending on the severity of the injury. The patient can be up and walking in the support but must not lift weights. Back exercises are essential.

SUBLUXATION & FRACTURES OF THE CERVICAL VERTEBRAE — WITHOUT NEUROLOGICAL SIGNS

These should be treated initially with a Glissons sling with 2-3 Kg weight over the head of the bed followed by skeletal skull traction for 3 — 6 weeks. Skull traction can be increased to about 4-10 Kg if necessary. After 3 weeks the patient is put in a Plastazote or skelecast collar for a further 6 to 9 weeks, depending on the severity of the injury.

A detachable collar of Plastazote or foam rubber is suitable for most patients.

FRACTURES OF THE SPINE
CLASSIFICATION
STABLE
(Intact Posterior Ligaments)

Transverse or   Wedge   Sacrum or   Burst
Spinous Process   Coccyx

USUALLY NO NEUROLOGICAL SIGNS EXCEPT BURST

UNSTABLE
(Ruptured Posterior Ligaments)

Atlas and   Cervical Spine   Thoracic or
Atlanto-Axial Joint   Lumbar

Dislocation or Fracture Dislocation   Severe Fracture or
Fracture Dislocation

MANY WITH NEUROLOGICAL SIGNS

OTHER SPINAL INJURIES
(X-rays May Appear Normal)

Spontaneous   Extension or   Prolapsed Disc
Reduction   Flexion   or
Before X-rays   Subluxation   Ligaments

ALL MAY DAMAGE SPINAL CORD

STABLE FRACTURES OF THE SPINE

TREATMENT

3 Days to 3 weeks
in Hospital

BACK EXERCISES

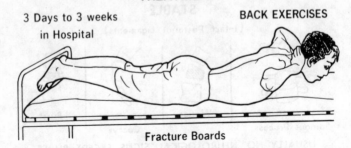

Fracture Boards

SPINAL SUPPORTS
Only in Severe or Multiple Fractures

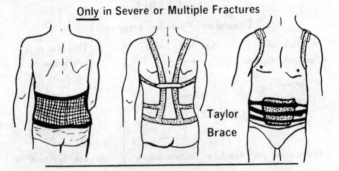

Taylor
Brace

FURTHER MANAGEMENT

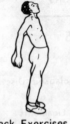

Back Exercises
Continued

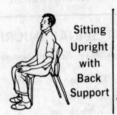

Sitting
Upright
with
Back
Support

Education

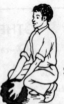

Lifting
with
Back
Straight

Avoiding Back Strain

STABLE FRACTURES OF THE SPINE

STABLE

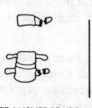

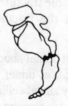

No
Displacement

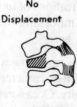

Intact
Supra
and
Inter
Spinous
Ligaments

**TRANSVERSE OR
SPINOUS PROCESS**

**SACRUM OR
COCCYX**

**THORACIC AND
LUMBAR SPINE**

CLINICAL EXAMINATION

NORMAL POWER

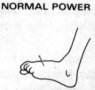

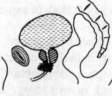

**NORMAL
SENSATION**

**NORMAL
REFLEXES**

**NORMAL BLADDER
AND RECTUM**

ASSOCIATED INJURIES

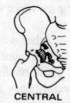

CALCANEUS

**CENTRAL
DISLOCATION OF HIP**

**OTHER SPINAL
FRACTURES**

COMPLICATIONS OF UNSTABLE FRACTURES OF SPINE

The complications of unstable fractures of the spine are often much more important than the fracture itself. The 3 main complications are:-

Bladder: In the early stages of spinal shock, there is retention of urine. **Intermittent** catheterisation under full sterile precautions may be necessary. Occasionally an indwelling catheter of polythene tubing or a plastic Foley catheter may be required.

Any indwelling catheter should usually be clamped, the clamp being released at about four-hourly intervals. This is to allow the bladder to maintain its tone. In some cases, however, continuous drainage is indicated.

A suprapubic catheter should **never** be inserted for neurological bladders. It leads to a small, contracted, infected bladder, ascending pyelitis and death. A fine suprapubic polythene tube may sometimes be indicated.

Any indwelling catheter should be removed at about 10 days and attempts made to obtain reflex emptying. This may, however, take a week or two longer to achieve and is usually much easier to achieve if **no** catheter has been inserted. An atonic bladder is a lower motor neurone type bladder and is partially emptied by suprapubic pressure. A reflex bladder is an upper motor neurone type bladder, and complete emptying is achieved by a spinal reflex often achieved by stimulating the inner side of the thigh or lower abdomen.

A soluble sulphonamide, or other suitable antibiotic should be given prophylactically for at least a month to prevent urinary tract infection, wherever there is a risk of this. Urinary retention and infection associated with recumbency may particularly lead to bladder or renal calculi. These usually occur in infected alkaline urine, are made of calcium ammonium phosphate and are radio opaque. They are fairly soft and when they take on the shape of the renal calices they are called stag horn calculi.

FRACTURES OF THE SPINE
EMERGENCY ASSESSMENT
SPINE

Palpate Tender Areas and Gaps Between Spinous Processes

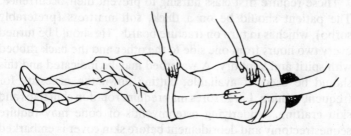

Roll Patient on Side   Do NOT Ever Sit Up
or Flex Spine

NEUROLOGICAL SIGNS

Respiration   Bladder   Sensation

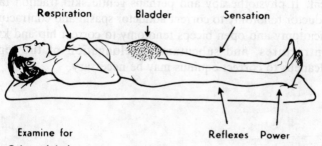

Examine for
Other Injuries
X-rays ONLY if Fit
Keep Patient Flat

Reflexes Power

The treatment of large calculi may mean removal, plus the management of the back pressure which caused the infection. In some cases this will entail endoscopic transurethral incision of the urethral sphincter.

BED SORES

These require first class nursing to prevent their occurrence. The patient should be on a thick, soft mattress (preferably sorbo), which is in turn on fracture boards. He should be turned every two hours from one side to the other and the back rubbed with spirit and kept dry. A waterbed may be indicated and this should be used, if available, cutting down the necessity for frequent turning. Large sores may require rotation skin flaps and skin grafting. Underlying osteomyelitis of bone may require sequestrectomy and debridement before skin cover is embarked upon.

CONTRACTURES

All paralysed limbs should be moved at least once a day through their full range of normal movement. Once contractures have developed, they can be very difficult, if not impossible, to treat. If physiotherapy and perhaps gentle skin traction fails, adductor tenotomy to correct adductor spasm and contracture, fasciotomy and open biceps tenotomy to correct hip and knee contractures, and subcutaneous elongation of the tendo calcaneus to correct equinus may be necessary.

SENSORY LEVELS

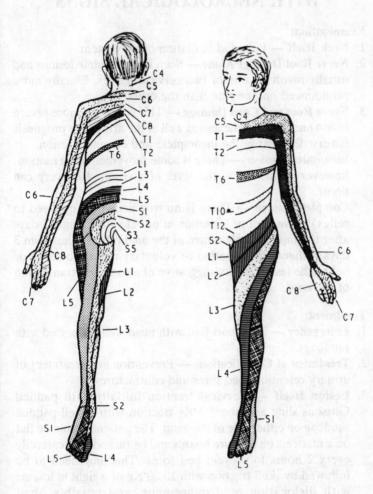

FRACTURES OF THE CERVICAL SPINE WITH NEUROLOGICAL SIGNS

Examination:
1. **Neck Itself** — Pain and limitation of movement.
2. **Nerve Root Damage Alone** — Seen in incomplete lesions and usually involving one or two cervical nerves. Usually more pronounced on one side than the other.
3. **Nerve Root and Cord Damage** — This is a much more severe lesion and involves the legs as well as the arms. The prognosis is very different in the incomplete and complete lesion.

    Incomplete Lesion — There is some movement or sensation, however slight, below the level of division. Recovery can occur.

    Complete Lesion — There is no true active (as opposed to reflex) movement or sensation at or below the lesion 3 days after the injury. Early return of the anal reflex in less than 3 days **without** any sensation or voluntary motor power at or below the lesion is very suggestive of a complete transection of the cord.

Treatment:
1. **Emergency** — Transport flat, with head well supported with sandbags.
2. **Treatment of Complications** — Prevention and treatment of urinary retention, bed sores and contractures.
3. **Lesion Itself** — Cervical traction **initially** with padded Glissons sling and about 3 Kg traction with a well padded sandbag on either side of the head. The patient should be flat on a mattress on fracture boards and be turned very carefully every 2 hours to prevent bed sores. This may need to be followed by skull traction with 10-20 Kg of weight in lesions with dislocation or displacement, and possibly open reduction.
4. **Progressive Lesion** — If deterioration occurs, an **urgent** myelogram followed by exploration is indicated.

FRACTURES OF THE CERVICAL SPINE

MOTOR EXAMINATION

Complete Transection of Cord

Paralysis Diaphragm	Complete Flaccid Paralysis

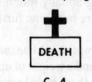

DEATH

C. 4.

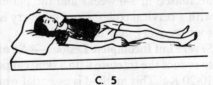

C. 5

Abduction Flexion Supination	Adduction Pronation
C. 6.	C. 7.
C. 5. Root Irritation	C. 6. Root Irritation

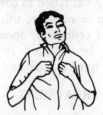

Paralysis Small Muscles of Hand

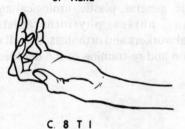

C. 8 T I

BELOW LESION

Complete Motor +
Sensory Paralysis +
Positive Anal Reflex

= Bad Prognosis
after 3 days.

5. **Unstable Fractures** — Fractures which are still unstable 8 weeks after injury should be stabilised by operation.
6. **Nerve Damage Alone** — Traction is maintained for 3 to 6 weeks and the patient then mobilised in a Minerva skelecast.
7. **Complete Lesion with No Recovery at All** — The traction is decreased in 3-6 weeks and the patient gradually mobilised with a cervical collar. Cord recovery is rare but some further root recovery may occur.
8. **Severe but Incomplete Lesions** — An attempt should be made to reduce the fracture with a skull caliper and a weight of up to 10-20 Kg. This method is essential where there is dislocation of one or both spinal facets, or where traction with a Glisson's sling has failed to correct displacement.

   In cases where this fails, or where redisplacement occurs after reduction, open reduction and wiring of the laminae may be indicated. In unstable dislocations bone grafting of the spine is indicated.

LATE TREATMENT

Support by plaster or plastic collar is required for at least 3 months from the time of the injury in all but the complete lesions. The late treatment of the quadraplegic patient with a complete lesion and **no recovery at all** is discussed under rehabilitation. This, however, must be planned **immediately** following an injury, as considerable psychological and social consequences result from permanent paralysis. A team effort is required whose members include orthopaedic, general, plastic, urological and neurosurgeons, physicians, nurses, physiotherapists, occupational therapists, social workers and orthotists, as well as specialists in the rehabilitation and re-training of the disabled.

CERVICAL SPINE

FRACTURES AND DISLOCATIONS

| CRUSH FRACTURE | ODONTOID PEG | FRACTURE DISLOCATION |

A/P Lateral and Oblique X-rays

EXAMINATION

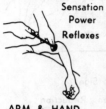

Sensation
Power
Reflexes

RESPIRATION

TRUNK AND

LOWER LIMB

ARM & HAND   BLADDER

INITIAL TREATMENT

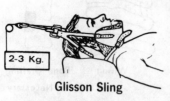 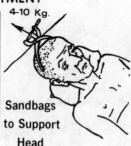

2-3 Kg.

4-10 Kg.

Glisson Sling

Head of Bed Elevated

**Sandbags
to Support
Head**

Fracture Boards WELL Padded Mattress

CERVICAL SPINE
FRACTURES AND DISLOCATIONS
MINOR STABLE INJURIES
No Neurological Signs

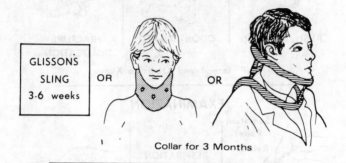

GLISSON'S
SLING
3-6 weeks

OR

OR

Collar for 3 Months

MAJOR INJURIES
With or Without Neurological Signs

7-15 Kg.
initially

Open Reduction
<u>Only</u> if Necessary

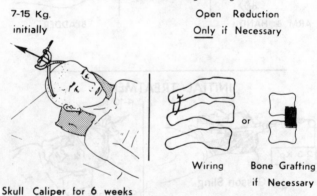

Skull Caliper for 6 weeks

Wiring

Bone Grafting
if Necessary

AVOID
Bed Sores
Contractures
Respiratory & Bladder Complications

CERVICAL SPINE
FURTHER TREATMENT

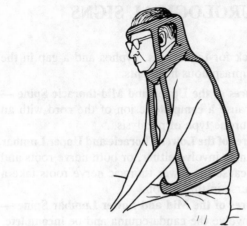

Skelecast up to 3 Months

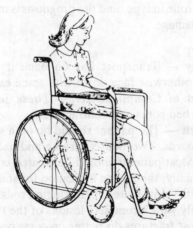

Padded Wheel Chair Complete Lesions

FRACTURES OF THE THORACIC AND LUMBAR SPINE WITH NEUROLOGICAL SIGNS

EXAMINATION

Examine the back for tenderness, kyphos and a gap in the interspinous and supraspinous ligaments.

1. **Unstable Fractures of the Upper and Mid-thoracic Spine —** These tend to cause a **complete** lesion of the cord with an upper motor neurone type of paralysis.

2. **Unstable Fractures of the Lower Thoracic and Upper Lumbar Spine —** These may involve either, or both nerve roots and cord. This is because the lower thoracic nerve roots take a very oblique course in this region.

3. **Unstable Fractures of the Mid and Lower Lumbar Spine —** These tend to involve the cauda equina and be **incomplete.** Recovery can occur to some extent. The paralysis is lower motor neurone in type, and the prognosis is much better than the cord damage.

TREATMENT

1. **Emergency —** Transport flat on back if possible, on a stretcher; otherwise face down with spine extended.

2. **Treatment of Complications —** These include urinary retention, bed sores and contractures.

3. **Lesion Itself —** The patient should be on a soft mattress on fracture boards. Two-hourly turning and back exercises are essential. Most patients should be treated conservatively.

   Occasionally, there is an indication for stabilisation of the fracture with spinal plates or Harrington rods. This should be done mainly with **incomplete** lesions of the thoraco- lumbar region. Most fractures do better on conservative treatment, but stabilisation may make for ease of nursing and earlier mobilisation. Some cauda equina lesions should be explored if pressure by disc or bone is suspected, but this is **not** indicated as a routine.

FRACTURES OF THE SPINE

UNSTABLE AND MAJOR THORACIC AND LUMBAR

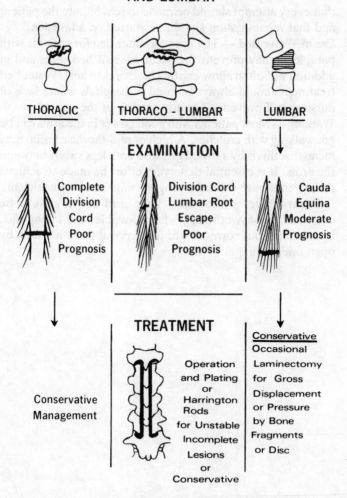

THORACIC | **THORACO - LUMBAR** | **LUMBAR**

EXAMINATION

Complete Division Cord Poor Prognosis	Division Cord Lumbar Root Escape Poor Prognosis	Cauda Equina Moderate Prognosis

TREATMENT

Conservative Management

Operation and Plating or Harrington Rods for Unstable Incomplete Lesions or Conservative

<u>Conservative</u>
Occasional Laminectomy for Gross Displacement or Pressure by Bone Fragments or Disc

4. **Progressive Lesions** — All lesions which are progressive should be explored as soon as possible.

5. **Late Treatment** — The patient should be mobilised in 8 to 12 weeks with the help of calipers and crutches. It is essential that every attempt should be made to rehabilitate the patient and that rehabilitation should be started **on admission.**

6. **Use of Water Bed** — The use of a water bed for patients with paraplegia may prevent the occurrence of bed sores and in addition will often allow existing bed sores to heal. Water bed treatment should always be used in hospitals where lack of nursing staff prevents 2-hourly turning of the patient.

7. **Walking** — Most patients with good power in the arms can be got walking with crutches. A high or mid-thoracic lesion may mean that this is by a tripod gait with both legs swung between the arms. It is essential that every effort be made to achieve this, even though ordinary progress might be by wheelchair.

Contractures of the hip, knee and ankle should be corrected by physiotherapy where possible, and failing this, by subcutaneous correction as far as possible, rather than by open operation.

FRACTURES OF THE SPINE

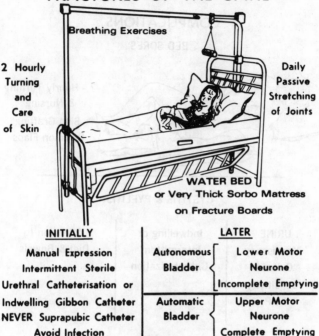

Breathing Exercises

2 Hourly Turning and Care of Skin

Daily Passive Stretching of Joints

WATER BED
or Very Thick Sorbo Mattress
on Fracture Boards

INITIALLY	LATER	
Manual Expression	Autonomous Bladder	Lower Motor Neurone Incomplete Emptying
Intermittent Sterile Urethral Catheterisation or Indwelling Gibbon Catheter		
NEVER Suprapubic Catheter Avoid Infection	Automatic Bladder	Upper Motor Neurone Complete Emptying

MOBILISATION

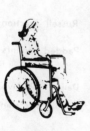

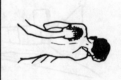

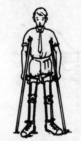

Wheel Chair

Crutches & Calipers

Training in Care of Bladder and Skin

FRACTURES OF THE SPINE

COMPLICATIONS

BED SORES

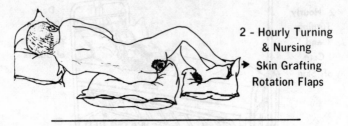

2 - Hourly Turning
& Nursing

Skin Grafting

Rotation Flaps

CYSTITIS & PYELITIS

URINE	Indwelling or	Attention to
Microscopy	Intermittent	Diet & Bowels
Culture	Catheterization	
Sensitivity		
I.V.P.		

CONTRACTURES

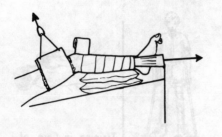

Russell Traction

Padded Splints

Daily Passive
Stretching

REHABILITATION
INITIAL TRAINING IN BED

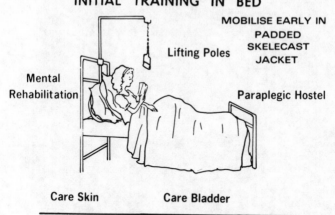

MOBILISE EARLY IN
PADDED
SKELECAST
JACKET

Lifting Poles

Mental
Rehabilitation

Paraplegic Hostel

Care Skin   Care Bladder

SOCIAL REHABILITATION

Aids to Daily Living

TRAINING FOR FUTURE EMPLOYMENT

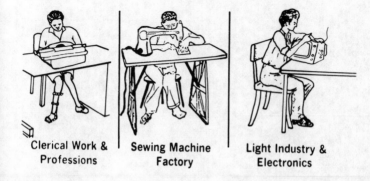

Clerical Work &
Professions

Sewing Machine
Factory

Light Industry &
Electronics

PELVIS

FRACTURES OF THE PELVIC RING CLASSIFICATION

MINOR FRACTURES
1. Isolated Chip off Iliac Crest
2. Fracture of Sacrum or Coccyx
3. Single Stable Fracture through Pelvic Ring

MAJOR FRACTURES
1. Anterior/Posterior Force
2. Vertical Force Fracture
3. Book Fracture

FRACTURE OF ACETABULUM
1. Minor
2. Major
3. Associated with Dislocation of Hip

COMPLICATIONS
1. **Sciatic Nerve**
   Neurapraxia — Common
   Axonotmesis — Common
   Neurotmesis — Rare
2. **Bladder Damage** (Common)
   Intraperitoneal Rupture
   Extraperitoneal Rupture
   Rupture Membranous Urethra
3. **Intestinal Damage** (Rare)
   Small Intestine
   Large Intestine
   Rectum
4. **Paralytic Ileus** (Common)
5. **Vascular Damage**

FRACTURES OF THE PELVIS

MINOR FRACTURES

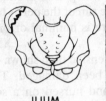 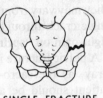

ILIUM | SINGLE FRACTURE PUBIS | SINGLE FRACTURE RING PELVIS (STABLE)

EXAMINATION

STABILITY OF PELVIC RING

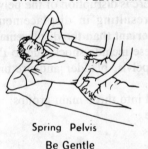

Spring Pelvis
Be Gentle

COMPLICATIONS

Damage ⟵ Bladder and Urethra

Sciatic Nerve

Vascular

Rectum and Anus

TREATMENT

Mattress on Fracture Boards for 3 days - 3 weeks	Leg Exercises and Early Walking

FRACTURES OF PELVIS
MINOR FRACTURES

These are fractures in which the "pelvic ring" is still stable. They may vary from an isolated chip off the rim of the pelvis to a **single** crack through the pelvic ring. There is minimal or only **slight** pain on **"springing"** the pelvis.

A pelvic fracture may be much more extensive than shown on x-ray, as the sacro-iliac joint may have been damaged. The patient should be admitted to hospital and nursed on a soft mattress, which is in turn on fracture boards. The patient can often be mobilised and discharged (with or without crutches) from one to three weeks after admission and often earlier, provided the sacro-iliac joint is not damaged.

MAJOR FRACTURES

These are fractures in which there is disruption of the pelvic ring in more than one place, resulting in displacement. Complications are **often more important than the displacement** itself and must be looked for. These include shock due to the considerable blood loss into the pelvis, bladder and urethral injuries, and sciatic nerve damage.

These fractures can be classified into three main groups:
1. Anterior/Posterior Force
2. Vertical Force
3. "Book" Fractures

In addition, fractures of the acetabulum may occur and these are discussed separately under "Dislocation of the Hip".

MAJOR FRACTURES OF THE PELVIS

CLASSIFICATION

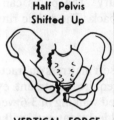 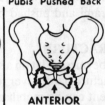 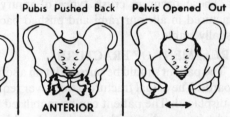

Half Pelvis Shifted Up	Pubis Pushed Back	Pelvis Opened Out
	ANTERIOR	
VERTICAL FORCE	POSTERIOR FORCE	"BOOK" FRACTURES

COMBINATIONS OF THESE MAY OCCUR

METHODS OF CAUSATION

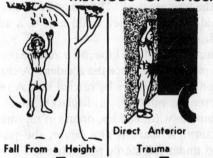 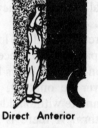 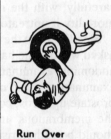

Fall From a Height	Direct Anterior Trauma	Run Over

COMMON COMPLICATIONS

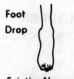 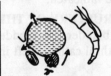

Foot Drop
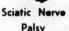

Sciatic Nerve Palsy	Rupture Bladder or Urethra	Pelvic Haematoma Rectum and Anus

FOR ACETABULAR FRACTURES SEE DISLOCATION OF HIP

ANTERIOR — POSTERIOR FORCE FRACTURES OF PELVIS

These occur in crush types of injury. The pubis can be fractured in all four rami and pushed back. The pelvic ring is usually stable.

TREATMENT OF FRACTURE

The patient should be nursed flat on a soft mattress on fracture boards. The actual fracture hardly ever requires treatment, even if displaced. The patient can be mobilised walking in 3-6 weeks and often earlier with crutches. In elderly patients without complications, the patient can often be mobilised in a few days.

URINARY COMPLICATIONS

The bladder and urethral complications of this fracture are far more important than the fracture itself. They must be looked for carefully, with the realisation that they could lead to a 100% mortality if untreated.

Bleeding from the urethra should be looked for and the patient asked whether he has passed urine since the accident. A careful abdominal examination should always be carried out. A rectal examination must **never** be omitted, as displacement of the prostate upwards, complete with bladder, occurs in ruptures of the membranous urethra. If there is any doubt, the patient should be catheterised under **full** sterile precautions.

A cystogram and an intravenous pyelogram should always be performed if there is any doubt about urinary tract damage. A urethogram may also be indicated.

INTRAPERITONEAL RUPTURE OF THE BLADDER

This occurs with a full bladder. The bladder should be repaired in two layers and a urethral catheter left in.

FRACTURES OF THE PELVIS
ANTERIOR-POSTERIOR FORCE

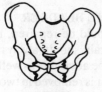 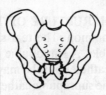

| MINIMAL DISPLACEMENT | MODERATE DISPLACEMENT PUBIS WITHOUT OTHER FRACTURES | FRACTURE PUBIS WITH DISRUPTION PELVIS |

TREATMENT
PUBIS ALONE
No Treatment for Displaced Pubis Itself

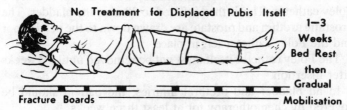

1–3 Weeks Bed Rest then Gradual Mobilisation

Fracture Boards

DISRUPTION PELVIS

Manipulation if Necessary

Traction for Upward Displacement

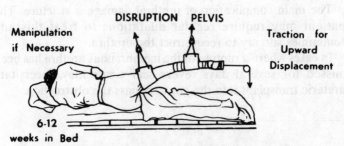

6-12 weeks in Bed

Displaced Pubis Manipulated Only if Bladder Requires Operation

TREAT COMPLICATIONS URGENTLY

In the case of severe bleeding or damage it is safer to leave in a suprapubic catheter or fine plastic tube as well for 2-3 days to help with bladder irrigation. The urethral catheter is removed after about two weeks.

EXTRAPERITONEAL RUPTURE OF THE BLADDER

This is relatively common. The tear should be repaired, but this is not often possible. A suprapubic drain should always be left in. A suprapubic catheter or tube may be advisable as well as a urethral catheter. The suprapubic catheter is removed in two or three days and the urethral catheter in two to three weeks.

RUPTURE OF THE MEMBRANOUS URETHRA

This is sometimes missed. The importance of a routine rectal examination in all fractures of the pelvis has already been mentioned.

The rupture is treated by opening the bladder and passing a metal sound into the prostatic urethra, as illustrated, to insert a Foley catheter. This is then inflated to 30ml in the bladder. The prostatic urethra and prostate are drawn down to the pelvic floor and the Foley catheter left in place.

The Foley catheter itself must **not** be removed until 2-3 weeks after insertion.

In all bladder and urethral injuries, the patient should be covered by chemotherapy for at least three weeks.

The main complication of urethral damage is stricture. The patient may require regular dilatations to treat this and sometimes surgery to reconstruct the urethra.

In cases where a rupture of the membranous urethra has been missed for several days severe scar tissue may necessitate ureteric transplant into the gut to bypass the obstruction.

FRACTURES OF THE PELVIS

COMPLICATIONS

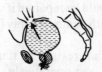

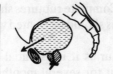

INTRAPERITONEAL
RUPTURE BLADDER

EXTRAPERITONEAL
RUPTURE BLADDER

RUPTURE
MEMBRANOUS
URETHRA

Treatment Described in Emergency Section

DAMAGE TO SCIATIC NERVE

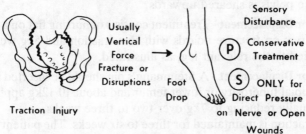

Usually
Vertical
Force
Fracture or
Disruptions

Traction Injury

Foot
Drop

Sensory
Disturbance

(P) Conservative
Treatment

(S) ONLY for
Direct Pressure
on Nerve or Open
Wounds

OTHER COMPLICATIONS

SHOCK
ANAEMIA

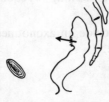

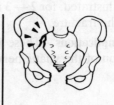

Vascular
Damage (S)

Rectum and
Colon Anus (S)

Late Pain in
"Book" Fracture (P)

RUPTURE OF THE PENILE URETHRA

If a partial or complete rupture is suspected a soft catheter should be passed with **full sterile precautions.** A urethogram is often of assistance. Complete ruptures should be repaired if seen early. Partial ruptures should be treated with a catheter only for 2 to 3 weeks.

In all urethral injuries it is essential that regular dilatation should be carried out for several months post-operatively.

VERTICAL FORCE
FRACTURES OF PELVIS

These are due to a fall from a height and the whole of one half of the pelvis is sheared upwards.

Minor Displacement - Treatment consists of nursing flat on a soft mattress on fracture boards with skin traction and 5kg weight applied to the relevant leg, as illustrated.

Major Displacement - A Steinmann's pin should be inserted into the tibial tuberosity or lower femur and about 10-12kg applied, gradually reducing to 7kg over two to three weeks.

Traction is maintained for three to six weeks. The patient can then be mobilised on crutches, but no weight bearing should be allowed on the affected side for two months after injury.

In very severe displacements of the pelvis an external fixateur, as illustrated, for 2 — 3 months may be required after reduction of the fracture.

Complications - These include an axonotmesis or a stretching lesion of the sciatic nerve.

FRACTURES OF THE PELVIS
VERTICAL FORCE

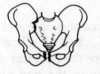

SLIGHT UPWARD DISPLACEMENT

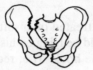

MODERATE OR MARKED DISPLACEMENT

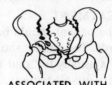

ASSOCIATED WITH CENTRAL DISLOCATION OF HIP

TREATMENT
SLIGHT DISPLACEMENT

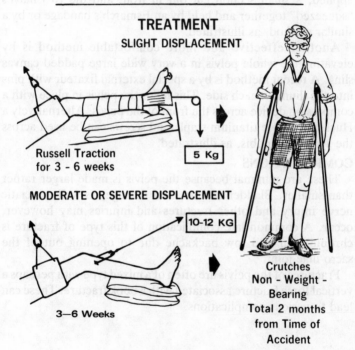

Russell Traction for 3 - 6 weeks

5 Kg

MODERATE OR SEVERE DISPLACEMENT

10-12 KG

3—6 Weeks

**Crutches
Non - Weight -
Bearing
Total 2 months
from Time of
Accident**

TREAT COMPLICATIONS AND SHOCK

'BOOK' FRACTURES OF PELVIS

In this the whole pelvis opens out like a book. The diastasis is usually, but not always, at the symphysis pubis.

TREATMENT

The patient should be treated on a soft mattress on fracture boards. The patient should be lying on his side and the effect of this is usually to "shut the book" (i.e. reduce the fracture). In severe displacement, a short anaesthetic in the bed and manipulation will usually achieve this adequately. In cases where this is not effective, a well padded plaster spica should be applied, a small section cut out in front and the two halves "squeezed" together and held by an Esmarch's bandage or by a similar method, as illustrated.

Another effective and more comfortable method is by elevating the whole pelvis in a very wide large padded canvas sling. A recent method is by a special external fixateur with pins into the ilium on each side. This holds the pelvis in place with a compression device across the front of the pelvis. Alternatively a Huckstep 2 hole titanium staple and screws can be used across the symphysis pubis, as illustrated.

COMPLICATIONS

These are minimal because the pelvis is made larger rather than smaller. Bladder and urethral damage, as well as sciatic nerve injury and other fractures and injuries may however, occur. A common late complication of this type of fracture is chronic pain and low backache due to opening out of the sacro-iliac joint.

Fractures of the pelvis are often of a mixed type with perhaps a vertical force fracture associated with a book fracture. These can lead to various complications.

FRACTURES OF THE PELVIS
BOOK FRACTURE

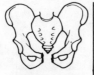 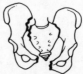

SYMPHYSIS PUBIS OPENED OUT **PUBIS FRACTURED** **ASSOCIATED WITH UPWARD DISPLACEMENT OF PELVIS**

TREATMENT

MINOR DISPLACEMENT
NO TREATMENT EXCEPT BED REST AND EARLY MOVEMENT

MAJOR DISPLACEMENT

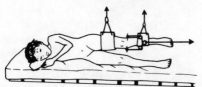

Traction for Upward Displacement of Pelvis

Fracture Boards   Manipulate under Anaesthetic if necessary
Patient in Bed 3-9 weeks
Upon Crutches Total of 3 Months

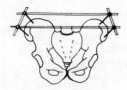

External Fixation for Unstable Fractures

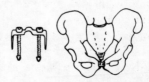

Huckstep 2 Hole Staple with Screws for Diastasis

LOWER LIMB

DISLOCATION OF THE HIP

1. Posterior

DISLOCATION OF THE HIP

CLASSIFICATION
1. Posterior
2. Anterior
3. Central

POSTERIOR DISLOCATION OF THE HIP

Diagnosis - The diagnosis is confirmed clinically by finding an extremely painful hip held in flexion, **adduction** and **internal** rotation. X-ray may show an associated fracture of the posterior rim of the acetabulum.

Reduction - Reduction is achieved by a good relaxant anaesthetic. The knee is flexed to a right angle and the hip externally rotated and lifted back into its socket. If not successful the patient should be on the floor to obtain added leverage.

The patient should be put into modified Russell traction for three to six weeks and kept **off** weight bearing for three months. Operative replacement with screw fixation may be required for a large displaced segment of the actabulum.

COMPLICATIONS

1. **Sciatic Nerve Damage** - This seldom requires operative interference unless a fracture of the acetabulum is causing pressure. In these cases operation is always required, together with screw replacement of the fragment.
2. **Avascular Necrosis of the Head of the Femur** - This will go on to osteoarthritis, which may require treatment. Technetium bone scanning is a useful investigation for diagnosing this early.
3. **Traumatic Ossification** - This should be treated by immobilisation in a skelecast spica in the early stages.

DISLOCATIONS OF THE HIP

ANTERIOR DISLOCATION	POSTERIOR DISLOCATION

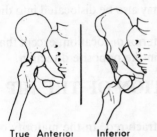 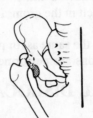

True Anterior	Inferior	Without Fracture Acetabulum	With Fracture Acetabulum

UNCOMMON	**COMMON**

EXAMINATION

ANTERIOR DISLOCATION	POSTERIOR DISLOCATION

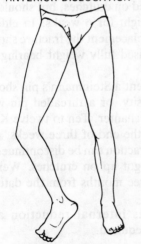 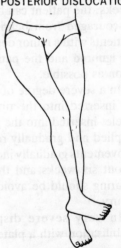

Abducted, Externally Rotated and Flexed	Adducted, Internally Rotated and Flexed

ANTERIOR DISLOCATION OF THE HIP

This is much less common than posterior dislocation.

The hip is abducted and externally rotated. The head of the femur may be felt in the groin. It may also be dislocated into the obturator fossa.

Treatment is the same as for posterior dislocation, except that the manipulations are performed in the opposite direction.

CENTRAL DISLOCATION OF THE HIP

The floor of the acetabulum is fractured. In the majority of cases the central displacement tends to be slight.

In slight degrees of displacement, treatment should be by skin traction with 4.5kg weight and a sling under the thigh with about 3kg weight (Russell traction modified). At the end of three weeks, the patient can be mobilised on crutches, but should be discouraged from bearing full weight for 6 weeks. In elderly patients with a minor degree of displacement the fracture should be **ignored** and the patient mobilised fully weight bearing, as soon as possible.

In a severe degree of displacement a Steinmann's pin should be inserted into the tibial tuberosity, or a threaded pin with eyelet inserted into the greater trochanter. Ten to twelve Kg is applied and gradually reduced at the end of three weeks, and movements gradually increased. Traction can be discontinued in about six weeks and the patient got up on crutches. Weight bearing should be avoided for three months from the date of injury.

In very severe displacements internal reduction and stabilisation with a plate may be required.

DISLOCATIONS OF THE HIP

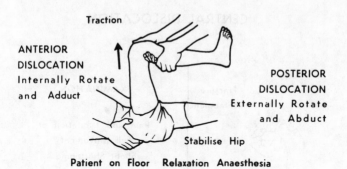

Traction

ANTERIOR DISLOCATION
Internally Rotate and Adduct

POSTERIOR DISLOCATION
Externally Rotate and Abduct

Stabilise Hip

Patient on Floor   Relaxation Anaesthesia

POST–REDUCTION

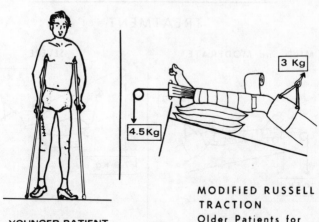

3 Kg

4.5 Kg

YOUNGER PATIENT -NON WEIGHT BEARING 3 MONTHS

OR

MODIFiED RUSSELL TRACTION
Older Patients for 3 Weeks Then Non–Weight-Bearing Crutches for 6 Weeks

DISLOCATIONS OF THE HIP

CENTRAL DISLOCATION

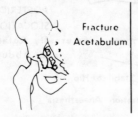

Fracture
Acetabulum

May be Associated with
Other Fractures of
the Pelvis

EXAMINATION

Pain and Limitation of
Full Movements
Slight Shortening

TREATMENT

MILD and MODERATE

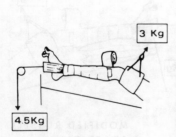

3 Kg

4.5Kg

MODIFIED RUSSELL
TRACTION for 1 - 6 Weeks
Then Non—Weight-Bearing
Crutches for 6 Weeks

SEVERE

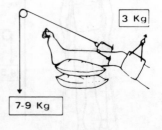

3 Kg

7-9 Kg

STEINMANN'S PIN for
4-6 Weeks Then
Modified Russell Traction
for 3-6 Weeks

DISLOCATIONS OF THE HIP

COMPLICATIONS

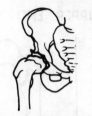

OSTEOARTHRITIS
All Types of Dislocation

**STIFFNESS and PAIN
IN HIP and KNEE**
All Types of Dislocation

**TOTAL HIP REPLACEMENT
SEVERE CASES**

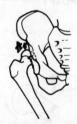

**EARLY RECURRENT
DISLOCATION**
Especially with
Acetabular Fractures

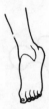

**SCIATIC NERVE
DAMAGE and FOOT DROP**
In Posterior Dislocation

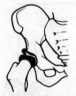

**AVASCULAR NECROSIS
HEAD OF FEMUR**
Anterior and Posterior Dislocation

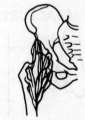

MYOSITIS OSSIFICANS

FRACTURES OF FEMUR

CLASSIFICATION

FRACTURES OF THE UPPER END

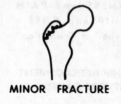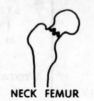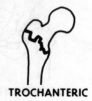

| MINOR FRACTURE | NECK FEMUR | TROCHANTERIC |

FRACTURES OF THE SHAFT

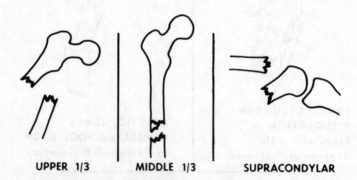

| UPPER 1/3 | MIDDLE 1/3 | SUPRACONDYLAR |

FRACTURES OF THE CONDYLES

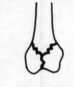

| ONE CONDYLE | T-SHAPED | COMMINUTED |

MINOR FRACTURES OF THE HIP
UPPER END OF FEMUR

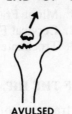
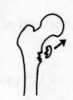

ISOLATED GREATER TROCHANTER

AVULSED GREATER TROCHANTER

AVULSED LESSER TROCHANTER

CAUSES

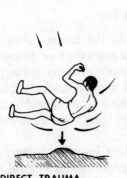
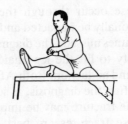

DIRECT TRAUMA

MUSCLE PULL IN ADOLESCENCE

TREATMENT

Bed Rest
Few Days Only → Crutches and
Physiotherapy → No
Complications

146

FRACTURES OF HIP

CLASSIFICATION
1. Minor Fractures
2. Cervical Fractures
3. Trochanteric Fractures

MINOR FRACTURES OF THE HIP

These include minor fractures of the greater and lesser trochanters. These fractures are small and isolated and do **not** extend through a major part of the femur. Treatment is by bed rest for a few days, followed by early mobilisation with crutches, if necessary, for up to three weeks.

CERVICAL FRACTURES OF THE HIP

These occur through the neck of the femur. They may occasionally be impacted and in these cases the true diagnosis is sometimes missed. The diagnosis is usually made by finding pain, inability to lift the leg unaided and marked external rotation (60°) and adduction. Both AP and lateral x-rays should be taken to confirm the diagnosis, as sometimes there is **no** displacement, and the fracture may be impacted.

These fractures are best treated by inserting compression screws, or blade plates under image intensifier control after reduction. Two or three Huckstep cannulated 6.5mm compression screws are particularly appropriate. Operative treatment is indicated because patients tend to be over 65 years of age. The complications of immobilising a patient of that age in bed in traction or a plaster spica are often bronchopneumonia, pulmonary embolus, venous thrombosis, urinary retention, bed sores, contractures and mental confusion.

Non-union of the neck, or avascular necrosis of the head of the femur, occurs in about one third of all cases.

FRACTURES OF NECK OF FEMUR

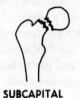 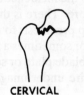 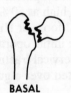

SUBCAPITAL | **CERVICAL** | **BASAL**

DIAGNOSIS

Pain, Inability to Lift Leg

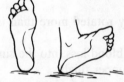

Foot Rotated Externally 60°

EXCEPTION
Impacted
Fracture

TREATMENT

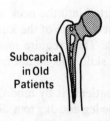 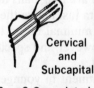 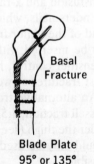

Subcapital in Old Patients

PROSTHESIS

Cervical and Subcapital

2 or 3 Cannulated Titanium Alloy 6·5mm Huckstep Compression Screws

Basal Fracture

Blade Plate 95° or 135°

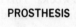

MOST OLD PATIENTS BEST TREATED BY PROSTHESIS AND IMMEDIATE FULL WEIGHT - BEARING

This condition does **not** always cause much pain and may require no operative treatment in old patients.

In subcapital fractures the incidence of avascular necrosis may be as high as 50% or more. There is therefore a very real place for a Moore or Huckstep prosthesis to replace the femoral head at the initial operation, or sometimes a total hip replacement. In low cervical fractures a blade plate or screw and plate should be inserted over a guide wire under image intensifier control.

TROCHANTERIC FRACTURES OF THE HIP

These occur through the trochanters and are usually comminuted. The same principles apply as for cervical fractures, with the following differences:-
1. The hip is usually externally rotated more than in cervical fractures (90°).
2. There may be considerable blood loss into the surrounding tissues with swelling of the upper thigh.
3. Non-union is uncommon.

Treatment is by a sliding screw and plate. This is a much larger operation than a compression screw and may require blood transfusion and x-ray control.

Enders nails, which are long nails inserted into the neck and head of the femur from just above the medial side of the knee, can be inserted with minimal blood loss. They require image intensifier control, however and specific skill, and do not hold most fractures as well.

An alternative treatment in younger patients is by modified Russell traction, 4.5kg skin traction on the leg and 3kg to a sling under the thigh (see illustration) for 8 — 12 weeks. This method should **only** be used where operation is contraindicated or not possible.

MAJOR TROCHANTERIC
FRACTURES OF FEMUR

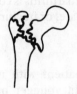

USUALLY COMMINUTED
Blood Loss ½ - 2 Litres

DIAGNOSIS

Pain, Shortening,
Inability to Lift Leg

**EXCEPTIONS
OCCUR**

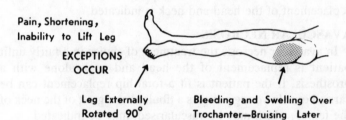

Leg Externally
Rotated 90°

Bleeding and Swelling Over
Trochanter—Bruising Later

TREATMENT

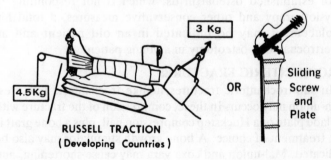

4.5 Kg

3 Kg

**RUSSELL TRACTION
(Developing Countries)**

OR

Sliding
Screw
and
Plate

COMPLICATIONS OF HIP FRACTURES

The complications of cervical fractures of the hip are mainly due to the poor blood supply of the head. This may cause non-union, or avascular necrosis. Late osteoarthritis is common. Penetration of the actebulum by a blade plate, or fracture of the nail or plate, can also occur.

NON-UNION

In **established** non-union in an old patient with minimal symptoms, no treatment is indicated. In younger patients, however, an intertrochanteric osteotomy is the treatment of choice, sometimes associated with a bone graft up the neck of the femur. In older patients a total hip replacement or prosthetic replacement of the head and neck is indicated.

AVASCULAR NECROSIS

In avascular necrosis the treatment of choice in a fairly unfit patient is replacement of the head and neck alone with a prosthesis. If the patient is fit a total hip replacement can be carried out. In young patients a fibular bone graft of the neck of the femur, which may be vascularised, may be indicated.

OSTEOARTHRITIS

In established osteoarthritis, which is not responding to physiotherapy and other conservative measures, a total hip replacement may be indicated in an old patient and an intertrochanteric osteotomy in a young patient.

TROCHANTERIC FRACTURES

In **sub**-trochanteric fractures, unlike trochanteric fractures, non-union may occur. In these, compression of the fracture with a blade plate or a Huckstep compression nail, plus a bone graft is the treatment of choice. A bone growth stimulator may also be indicated. Mal-union and coxa vara may cause shortening, and osteotomy and correction with a compression plate may be necessary if conservative measures fail.

COMPLICATIONS OF HIP FRACTURES

CERVICAL FRACTURES

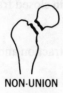

NON-UNION

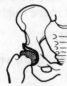

AVASCULAR NECROSIS

OSTEOARTHRITIS

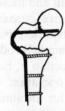

INTEROCHANTERIC OSTEOTOMY
<u>Not</u> if Old and Minimal Symptoms

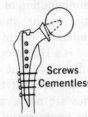

Screws
Cementless

HUCKSTEP CERAMIC AND TITANIUM HIP
Hemiarthroplasty or Total Hip

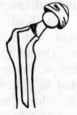

TOTAL HIP REPLACEMENT

TROCHANTERIC FRACTURES

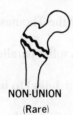

NON-UNION
(Rare)

MALFUNCTION + COXA VARA
(Common) ➡ **SHORTENING**

FRACTURES OF THE FEMORAL SHAFT

All patients require admission. Associated injuries must be watched for. The patient may be very shocked and 2 litres or more of blood may be lost in the thigh, even in closed fractures.

EMERGENCY TREATMENT

Use a well padded Thomas splint with skin traction and the leg straight. (See illustration).

SUBSEQUENT TREATMENT

Adults with severe comminution of the shaft and those in the lower one third of the femur, may require conservative treatment, with a Steinmann's pin in the tibial tuberosity and traction. The alternative is a Huckstep titanium nail and screws plus circlips. Conservative treatment with traction is, however, indicated in patients who are not fit for operation, and in hospitals where facilities are not available for intramedullary nailing. The subsequent treatment of these patients is divided into three stages in an adult:

FIRST STAGE — First Four Weeks Approximately.

1. The patient is in a Thomas splint with a Pearson's knee piece. The end of the Thomas splint and the knee piece are attached by cord so that the knee is at an angle of about 30°. (See illustration).
2. One cord is attached to the upper end of the Thomas splint with about 3kg pulling headwards.
3. One cord to the lower end of the Thomas splint parallel with cord (2).
   There should be just enough weight (about 3-4kg) to balance the leg in mid air.
4. Traction on the Steinmann's pin to the femur through a "modified" Bohler stirrup with 6-7kg and applied in the line of the femur.
5. Padded leather straps under the femur.

FRACTURE FEMUR

EMERGENCY TREATMENT

IMMOBILISE LIMB	STOP HAEMORRHAGE
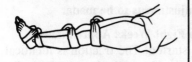	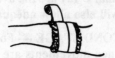
2 Legs Together or Thomas Splint	DIRECT PRESSURE TREAT OTHER INJURIES

TRANSPORT TO HOSPITAL

Thomas Splint if Available   Traction

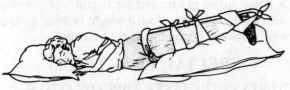

Foot of Stretcher Elevated

INITIAL TREATMENT IN HOSPITAL

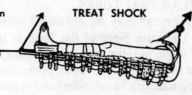

Skin Traction   TREAT SHOCK

Thomas Splint

Blood Transfusion and Other Treatment if Necessary

XRAY AND OTHER DEFINITIVE TREATMENT ONLY WHEN GENERAL CONDITION PERMITS

6. Intravenous pethidine in the ward may be necessary to obtain a good manipulative correction.

7. X-rays on about two occasions in the first two weeks. Thereafter one at four weeks, one at eight weeks and one final x- ray are the average. **Clinical measurement of the limb will also allow adequate adjustments to be made.**

SECOND STAGE — Four to Eight Weeks Approximately.

Knee movements are now started. The traction is identical, except that the Pearson's knee piece is attached to an extra pulley and weight so that the patient can now move his knee.

THIRD STAGE — Eight to Twelve Weeks Approximately.

When the fracture is clinically uniting, the patient can be mobilised further and the weight reduced. As soon as the x-rays are satisfactory, the Steinmann's pin is removed. A cast brace, which is a well fitting plaster cast for fractures of the middle or lower one third, will allow graded weight bearing on crutches. Otherwise mobilise, gradually weight bearing.

SPECIAL FRACTURES

FRACTURES IN THE UPPER THIRD OF FEMUR

The upper fragment is abducted and flexed by the hip muscles. The leg should be fully abducted to compensate for this. An intramedullary nail is probably the best method of treatment.

SUPRACONDYLAR FRACTURES

The lower fragment may be rotated backwards by the gastrocnemius. The knee piece of the Thomas splint must be flexed to a right angle to relax the gastrocnemius, with a pad of wool behind the lower fragment. Open operation with a blade plate or Huckstep nail may be necessary or a cylinder plaster, or skelecast with the knee well flexed.

DIFFICULT FRACTURES

A Kuntscher or Huckstep solid intramedullary nail with screw fixation may have to be used.

FRACTURES OF FEMORAL SHAFT
INITIAL SKELETAL TRACTION

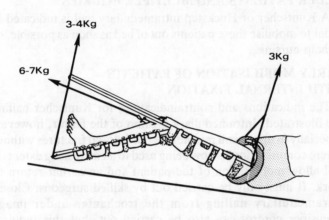

3-4Kg

6-7Kg

3Kg

HUCKSTEP THOMAS SPLINTS	HUCKSTEP BÖHLER STIRRUP

HUCKSTEP THOMAS SPLINTS

Adjustable Length and Ring

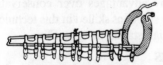

Split Ring + Padding

SINGLE SPLINT SUITABLE FOR ALL LIMBS AND BOTH SIDES

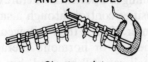

Shortened +
Pearson's Knee Piece

HUCKSTEP BÖHLER STIRRUP

Denham threaded Pin

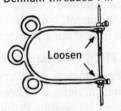

Loosen

PROCEDURE

Insert Denham Pin
Under G.A. or L.A.
Manipulate Fracture
Put up Traction in Theatre

In compound dirty fractures, external fixation with pins and a Wagner, or other type of fixateur, to correct angulation and shortening may be ideal.

OLDER PATIENTS AND MULTIPLE INJURIES

A Kuntscher or Huckstep intramedullary nail is indicated in order to mobilise these patients out of bed as soon as possible, or to help nursing.

EARLY MOBILISATION OF PATIENTS WITH INTERNAL FIXATION

The indications and contraindications for Kuntscher nailing are illustrated. Intramedullary fixation of the femur, however, especially in upper and middle one third closed fractures without severe comminution, is now being used to an increasing extent. It will allow mobilisation of the patient and an earlier return to work. It must only be carried out by skilled surgeons. Closed intramedullary nailing from the trochanter under image intensifier control can also be carried out, but this requires considerable skeletal traction in most cases, as well as experience with this method.

In summary, the treatment of **suitable** cases with open or closed intramedullary nailing has many advantages over conservative management, but **only** if done by surgeons skilled in this technique and in operating theatres with high standards of sterility.

PATHOLOGICAL FRACTURES

Pathological fractures are often due to secondary deposits from carcinoma. These should be treated before a fracture occurs, if possible. Prophylactic nailing of a **potential** fracture can be done easily under image intensifier control through a small incision above the greater trochanter. This is then followed by radiotherapy, adjuvant chemotherapy or hormone therapy. Once a fracture has occurred a nail can still be used, but the pathological area may need strengthening with methyl methacrylate cement to allow the patient early mobility after radiotherapy.

FRACTURES OF FEMORAL SHAFT

MOBILISATION OF KNEE

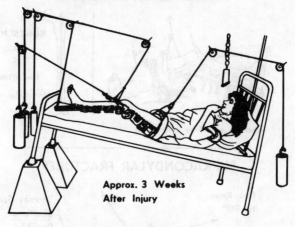

Approx. 3 Weeks
After Injury

ADDITIONAL TREATMENT

X-RAYS OR CLINICAL MEASUREMENT	PHYSIOTHERAPY and MOBILISATION
Initial Post–Reduction	Quadriceps Exercises + Adjustment of Sling } Daily
3 Days	
1 Week	Knee Movement on Traction — 3 Weeks
3 Weeks	
6 Weeks	Knee Movements Free in Bed } Good Callus 9-12 Weeks
9 Weeks	
3 Months	Up on Crutches { Bony Union 3 Months
6 Months	
	Full Weight-Bearing { Solid Union 4-6 Months

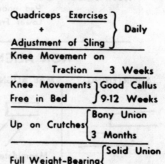

FRACTURES OF FEMORAL SHAFT

FRACTURES UPPER 1/3rd

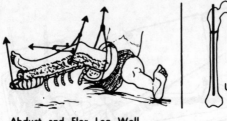

KÜNTSCHER
NAIL
if
Reduction
Unsatisfactory

Abduct and Flex Leg Well

SUPRACONDYLAR FRACTURES

Flex Knee
to 90°

Thomas Splint
Shortened if
Possible

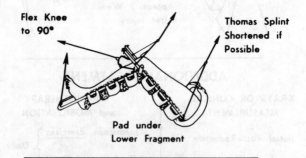

Pad under
Lower Fragment

NON ALIGNMENT

SHORTENING	MAL ALIGNMENT	SOFT TISSUE INTERPOSITION

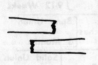

Increase Traction

Manipulate
in Bed G. A.

Internal Fixation

FRACTURES OF FEMORAL SHAFT

FEMUR PLUS TIBIA

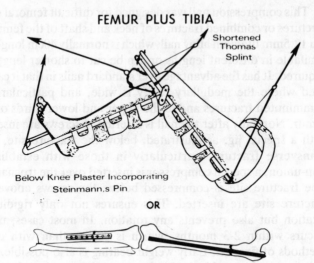

Shortened
Thomas
Splint

Below Knee Plaster Incorporating
Steinmann.s Pin

OR

Compression Plate Tibia plus Huckstep or Kuntscher Nail

KÜNTSCHER NAIL FEMUR

ABSOLUTE INDICATIONS	REL. CONTRAINDICATIONS
Pathological Fractures	Severe Compound Fractures
Mentally Confused Patients	Risk of Secondary Infection
Senile Patients	Fracture Lower 1/3rd
Associated Other Severe Injuries	Severely Comminuted Fractures
Soft Tissue Interposition	**USE**
Non-Union — Some Cases	**HUCKSTEP NAIL --**
Failed Conservative Treatment	**FOR** **DIFFICULT FRACTURES**

HUCKSTEP COMPRESSION NAIL

This compression nail was designed for difficult femoral shaft fractures or combined fractures of neck and shaft of the femur. It is a 12.5mm titanium alloy nail, which is normally 40cm long. It is available in different lengths or can be cut to shorter lengths if required. It has the advantage over standard nails in that it can be used where the medullary cavity is wide, and particularly in comminuted fractures and in the upper and lower thirds of the femur. Normally after the nail is inserted, 4 screws are inserted with a special jig, as illustrated, below the fracture site. In a transverse fracture, particularly in those with established non-union, a special compressor is inserted over the trochanter. The fracture site is compressed before the screws above the fracture site are inserted. This ensures not only rigidity of fixation but also prevents any rotation. In most cases, union occurs within 2-3 months, which is earlier than with other methods of fixation. Early weight bearing is also possible. The nail can also be used in double fractures of the neck and shaft of the femur, as one end of the nail has oblique holes which allow fixation of the neck with long lag screws.

The nail is particularly indicated in established non-union where rigidity of fixation and compression are required. In these cases bone grafting is usually used as well.

In comminuted fractures, or oblique fractures with a wide medullary cavity, the nail is used without compression. The nail has also been shown to be stronger than the average femoral shaft in four point bending torsion and tensile testing. A minimum of 3 screws below and above the fracture is also equivalent to the strength of the nail.

In femoral shortening the screws are inserted **above** the fracture site initially instead of below. The femur is lengthened before the lower screws are inserted. A bone graft is then applied.

HUCKSTEP INTRAMEDULLARY FEMORAL COMPRESSION NAIL
RIGID STRONG FIXATION WITH COMPRESSION

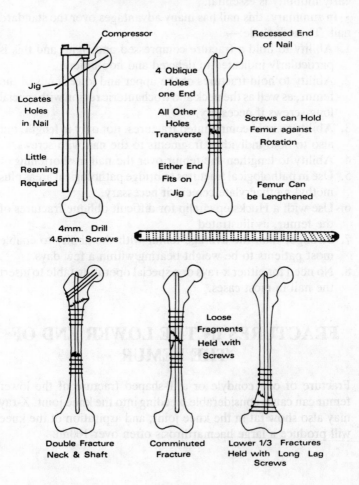

Compressor

Jig Locates Holes in Nail

Little Reaming Required

4mm. Drill
4.5mm. Screws

Recessed End of Nail

4 Oblique Holes one End

All Other Holes Transverse

Either End Fits on Jig

Screws can Hold Femur against Rotation

Femur Can be Lengthened

Double Fracture Neck & Shaft

Comminuted Fracture

Loose Fragments Held with Screws

Lower 1/3 Fractures Held with Long Lag Screws

This method of lengthening has proved to be very successful in several hundred cases and the nail is now being used, not only in non-union and in difficult fractures, but also in some cases where early mobility is essential.

In summary, this nail has many advantages over the standard nail. These include:—

1. Ability to hold a fracture compressed and rigid, and this is particularly indicated in delayed and non-union.
2. Ability to hold fractures of the upper and lower ends of the femur, as well as the neck and trochanteric region with special long screws if necessary.
3. Ability to hold comminuted fractures, not only **to length**, but also to hold individual fragments to the nail with screws.
4. Ability to lengthen the femur over the nail in shortening.
5. Use in pathological fractures to bridge pathological areas plus methyl methacrylate cement if necessary.
6. Use with a Huckstep circlip for difficult oblique fractures of the femur, as illustrated.
7. Stronger than the average femur with the ability to enable most patients to be weight bearing within a few days.
8. No need for either x-rays or a special operating table to insert the nail in most cases.

FRACTURES IN THE LOWER END OF THE FEMUR

Fracture of one condyle or a T-shaped fracture of the lower femur can cause considerable bleeding into the knee joint. X-ray may also show fat in the knee joint, and aspiration of the knee will produce a large haemarthrosis often over 100ml.

DIFFICULT FRACTURES
UPPER 1/3 rd FEMUR

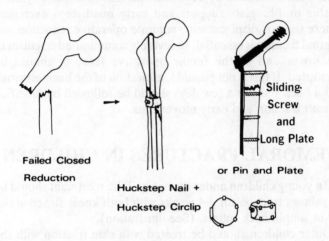

Failed Closed
Reduction

Huckstep Nail +
Huckstep Circlip

or Pin and Plate

Sliding
Screw
and
Long Plate

SUPRACONDYLAR FRACTURE

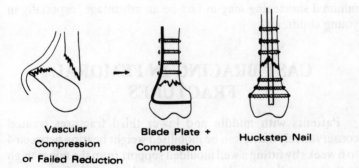

Vascular
Compression
or Failed Reduction

Blade Plate +
Compression

Huckstep Nail

In patients with minimal or no displacement treatment should be by aspiration under full sterile precautions, followed by a pressure bandage with wool and rest on a Thomas splint for a few days. This is followed by a cylinder skelecast, complete cylinder plaster or fibreglass support and early quadriceps exercises. Where there is displacement, accurate operative reduction and internal fixation is essential. In severely comminuted fractures of the lower end of the femur operative fixation should be attempted. If this is not possible, aspiration of the haemarthrosis and a back slab for a few days should be followed by modified Russell traction and early movements.

FEMORAL FRACTURES IN CHILDREN

In young children under the age of 3 the treatment should be by gallows traction for 3-4 weeks with both knees flexed about 10° in simple back splints. (See illustration).

Older children should be treated with **skin** traction with the knee straight, as illustrated, in a Thomas splint. Internal fixation should be avoided in children. There is commonly an overgrowth of the leg in children after fractures, and this is usually 1-2cm. It is important, therefore, that the leg is **not** over distracted, and minimal shortening may in fact be an advantage, especially in young children.

CAST BRACING IN FEMORAL FRACTURES

Patients with middle and lower third fractures treated conservatively may often be mobilised weight bearing between 4 to 6 weeks by fitting a well moulded support from the upper thigh to the toes with a knee hinge to prevent the last 20° of extension. This allows mobility of the knee while still preventing the rotation of the tibia being transmitted to the femoral shaft.

FRACTURES LOWER END OF FEMUR

CONDYLES AND T-FRACTURES

 OR

CONSERVATIVE   **OPERATIVE**

Aspirate
Blood and
Manipulate

Screw

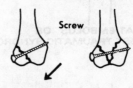

Padded Cylinder Plaster and
Non-Weight-Bearing for 2 Months

COMMINUTED

 → Aspirate Blood From Knee
Wool plus Crepe
Bandage for 3 Days

THEN

Skin Traction
+
Energetic Exercises
for 6 Weeks

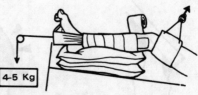

4–5 Kg

OR INTERNAL FIXATION

COMPLICATIONS OF FRACTURES
OF THE FEMORAL SHAFT

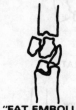

Comminuted Fractures

"FAT EMBOLUS" OR
POST TRAUMATIC SYNDROME

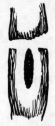

Compound Fractures and Infected Kuntscher Nails

OSTEOMYELITIS

Over Distraction

DELAYED and
NON-UNION

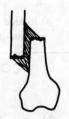

Inadequate Traction

SHORTENING

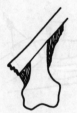

MAL UNION

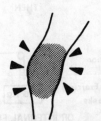

Inadequate Exercise Damage to Joint

PAIN, SWELLING
and STIFFNESS OF KNEE

FRACTURES OF THE LOWER END
OF FEMUR
COMPLICATIONS

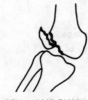

GENU VALGUM

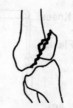

GENU VARUM

**PAIN, SWELLING
and STIFFNESS**

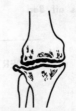

OSTEOARTHRITIS

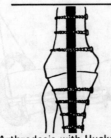

Arthrodesis with Huckstep
Compression Nail
or
External Compression Fixateur

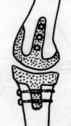

Huckstep Cementless
Ceramic Knee
with
Screw Fixation

FRACTURES OF FEMORAL SHAFT

FRACTURES IN CHILDREN

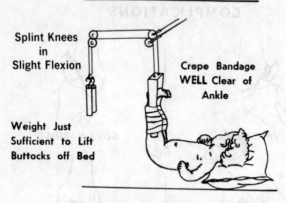

Splint Knees
in
Slight Flexion

Crepe Bandage
WELL Clear of
Ankle

Weight Just
Sufficient to Lift
Buttocks off Bed

UNDER 15Kg - GALLOWS TRACTION

Average 3 Weeks

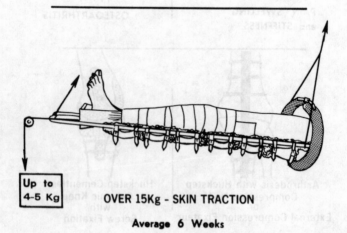

Up to
4-5 Kg

OVER 15Kg - SKIN TRACTION

Average 6 Weeks

CLASSIFICATION OF KNEE INJURIES
LIGAMENTOUS INJURIES

MEDIAL LIGAMENT
1. Sprain
2. Partial Rupture
3. Complete Rupture

LATERAL LIGAMENT
1. Sprain
2. Partial Rupture
3. Complete Rupture

ANTERIOR & POSTERIOR CRUCIATES
1. Without Rupture of Medial or Lateral Ligaments
2. One Cruciate + Medial or Lateral Ligament
3. Both Cruciates + Medial or Lateral Ligament

ISOLATED BONY INJURIES

PATELLA
1. Crack Fracture
2. Clean Separation
3. Comminution
4. Dislocated Patella

LOWER END FEMUR
1. One Condyle
2. T-shape both Condyles
3. Severely Comminuted Fracture

UPPER END TIBIA
(Plateau Fractures)
1. Minimal Displacement
2. Downward Displacement of Lateral Tibial Plateau
3. Crush Lateral Plateau

PATELLA

CRACK FRACTURE

This is due to direct trauma. There is no displacement and nearly always a haemarthrosis. Aspirate the haemarthrosis and apply a firm crepe bandage over wool for three days. Then apply cylinder plaster or skelecast for three to six weeks and carry out quadriceps exercises in all patients with a fracture.

CLEAN BREAK IN TWO

Usually caused by a sudden flexion strain. The patient is unable to hold his leg up straight against gravity, and there is swelling and often a palpable gap over the front of the patella. There is always a haemarthrosis. Excise the patella if the back of the patella is rough. In a clean break, a screw or wire can be used, as illustrated. The tension band wire with 2 Kirschner wires is best.

COMMINUTED FRACTURES

Caused by a direct fall on to the patella. Considerable swelling, tenderness and a haemarthrosis always occurs. Treatment is **always** by patellectomy followed by a plaster or skelecast for 6 weeks. This is because the rough back of the patella will cause osteoarthritis.

BIPARTITE PATELLA

This is a congenital abnormality, often with an apparent fracture, usually in the upper outer quadrant. The x-ray shows a well formed edge and examination shows lack of local tenderness. This abnormality may be present on the opposite side.

DISLOCATED PATELLA

This is commonly recurrent and is more common in girls with genu valgum. The knee gives way suddenly with severe pain. The patella is displaced laterally and can be reduced by straightening the knee. Operation may be required to prevent further recurrences.

FRACTURES OF THE PATELLA

CRACK FRACTURE
NO DISPLACEMENT

COMMINUTED
FRACTURE

CLEAN BREAK

CAUSES

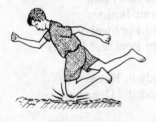
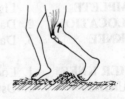

DIRECT TRAUMA

SUDDEN PULL ON
QUADRICEPS

TREATMENT

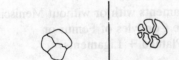
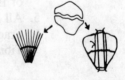

Aspirate Blood
Up to 14 Days
after Trauma

Excise
In all Cases
Except
Old Patients

Excise
In Patient over
30 or if Irregular
Posterior Surface

Screw or Wire
In Young
Patient

MISCELLANEOUS KNEE INJURIES

MENISCAL INJURIES
1. Injury Coronary Ligaments
2. Medial Meniscus
3. Lateral Meniscus

EXTENSOR MECHANISM KNEE
1. Ligamentum Patellae or Insertion
2. Separation of Patella
3. Tears of Quadriceps Mechanism

COMPLETE DISLOCATION OF KNEE
1. Associated Bony and Ligamentous Injuries
2. Damage to Popliteal Vessels
3. Damage to Popliteal Nerves

OTHER KNEE INJURIES
1. Loose Body in Knee
2. Osteochondritis Dissecans

COMBINED KNEE INJURIES
1. Medial Ligament + Medial Meniscus
2. Medial Ligament + Anterior Cruciate
3. Medial Ligament + Both Cruciates
4. Lateral Ligament + One or Both Cruciates
5. All Ligaments with or without Menisci
6. Fracture Condyles of Femur or Tibial Plateau + Ligaments

FRACTURES OF THE PATELLA

FURTHER TREATMENT

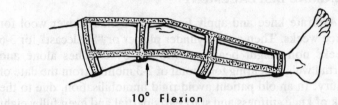

10° Flexion
of Knee

1" Below Groin

1" Above Medial
Malleolus

USE SKELECAST IF AVAILABLE

or

Cylinder Plaster

For Four Weeks

plus

Static Quadriceps Exercises

AFTER REMOVAL OF PLASTER

| Crepe Bandage | Energetic Quadriceps Exercises |

COMPLICATIONS

| Instability of Knee and Lack of Full Extension | Stiffness, Pain and Late Osteoarthritis |

UPPER END OF TIBIA
(Lateral Plateau Fractures)

MINIMAL DISPLACEMENT

Aspirate knee and apply firm crepe bandage over wool for three weeks. Then apply cylinder plaster or "Skelecast" for 3-6 weeks non-weight bearing, followed by crutches alone and partial weight bearing for a total of 2-3 months from the date of injury. In an old patient avoid rigid immobilisation, due to the risk of knee stiffness and start early partial and even full weight bearing and ignore the fracture. Give early quadriceps and mobilising exercises for the knee, plus a knee support.

DOWNWARD DISPLACEMENT
OF LATERAL TIBIAL PLATEAU

Aspirate knee and manipulate under general anaesthetic. Above-knee padded non-weight bearing plaster for three months. If manipulation fails **open** reduction with screw fixation plus bone graft from the lower femur.

SEVERE CRUSH OF LATERAL PLATEAU

Aspirate haemarthrosis, plus a firm pressure bandage over wool, plus Russell traction. Quadriceps and knee exercises are started the day after injury and maintained for six weeks. The patient is **non-weight** bearing for 2-3 months. Packing with bone graft under the fracture after reducing the displaced plateau is indicated in young patients with moderate or severe crush injuries.

COMPLICATIONS

These include pain, stiffness and recurrent effusion early. Later a valgus deformity with arthritis in the lateral compartment of the knee may occur, and this may require osteotomy or occasional total knee replacement.

KNEE INJURIES

FRACTURE TIBIAL PLATEAU

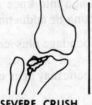
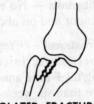

MINIMAL CRUSH **SEVERE CRUSH** **ISOLATED FRACTURE PLATEAU**

CAUSATION

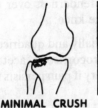

Bumper Fracture

IMMEDIATE TREATMENT

Crepe Bandage Over Wool   Aspirate Blood

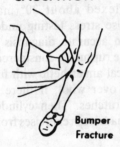

Examine for Medial Ligament Damage

FURTHER TREATMENT

MINIMAL CRUSH	SEVERE CRUSH	ISOLATED FRACTURE
Aspirate Blood	Russell Traction	Screw +
Crepe Bandage	for 6 Weeks	Bone Graft
Early Movements	or Bone Graft	if Necessary

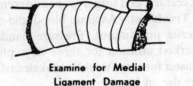

ENERGETIC QUADRICEPS EXERCISES
NON-WEIGHT BEARING – 2 MONTHS TOTAL

LIGAMENTOUS INJURIES OF KNEE

SPRAIN

Diagnosis — No effusion into knee, but tenderness over the ligament and on abducting or adducting the knee.

Treatment — Crepe bandage plus ice initially and quadriceps exercises. An injection of 1ml. of hydrocortisone acetate 25mg/ml + local anaesthetic may be necessary if pain persists for more than six weeks.

PARTIAL RUPTURE

Diagnosis - Usually effusion or haemarthrosis into knee. Tenderness and swelling over ligament and tender on abducting or adducting knee with the knee flexed about 30° may demonstrate laxity of the ligaments. Use stress testing under general anaesthetic with an x-ray if an accurate diagnosis is necessary, and surgery for early complete rupture is considered.

Treatment - Aspirate blood under local anaesthetic with full sterile precautions. Pressure bandage over wool, if there is marked effusion for three days plus crutches. Then cylinder plaster for three weeks or a skelecast. Quadriceps exercises from the **day** of injury.

COMPLETE RUPTURE

Diagnosis - There is usually a haemarthrosis. There is tenderness, swelling and laxity of the collateral ligaments. The anterior or posterior cruciates, or both, may also be ruptured and lax. **If in doubt** treat as a complete rupture.

Treatment - Admit patient to hospital. Aspirate blood. (Remains fluid for ten to fourteen days.) Then firm crepe pressure bandage over plenty of wool. Leg bandaged onto a Thomas splint for 3 days. Then cylinder plaster or skelecast for 6 weeks. Static quadriceps exercises from day after injury.

LIGAMENTOUS INJURIES OF THE KNEE

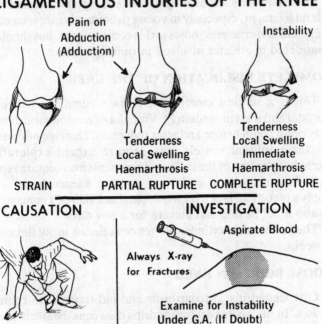

Pain on Abduction (Adduction)

Instability

STRAIN

PARTIAL RUPTURE
Tenderness
Local Swelling
Haemarthrosis

COMPLETE RUPTURE
Tenderness
Local Swelling
Immediate
Haemarthrosis

CAUSATION

INVESTIGATION

Aspirate Blood

Always X-ray for Fractures

Examine for Instability Under G.A. (If Doubt)

TREATMENT

Partial or Complete Rupture

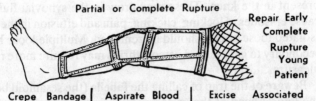

Repair Early
Complete
Rupture
Young
Patient

Crepe Bandage
Strain Alone

Aspirate Blood
(Up to 2 weeks)

Excise Associated
Tear Medial Meniscus

CREPE BANDAGE + ENERGETIC QUADRICEPS EXERCISES
<u>SKELECAST</u> INSTEAD OF PLASTER IS BETTER

There is an indication for operation and repair of the medial or lateral ligament, especially in young patients who are seen early. Repair of the cruciates, however, is controversial, but should be considered in athletes involved in running sports.

COMPLETE DISLOCATION OF THE KNEE

This is a surgical emergency. Always admit the patient to hospital and treat immediately. Vascular or neurological damage may occur, both before and after reduction. Damage or pressure on the popliteal vessels may require urgent exploration. Complete rupture of the collateral ligaments may require repair.

Reduce dislocation early and aspirate haemarthosis. Then apply a crepe bandage over wool, plus back slab or Thomas splint in about 30° flexion and elevate for a few days.

Then a complete cylinder plaster or skelecast in 30° flexion for 6 weeks.

LOOSE BODIES IN KNEE

Osteochondritis, osteoarthritis and old trauma are common causes. In the case of osteochondritis dissecans the site is usually the lateral side of the medial condyle. Synovial fringes may be nipped, or fragments of damaged articular cartilage may be present in the knee. These may grow in the synovial fluid and cause episodes of locking, clicking, pain and effusion in the knee. Isolated loose bodies should be removed. Multiple loose bodies secondary to generalised osteoarthritis may require more radical measures.

Beware of the trap of calling the **fabella** (the sesamoid bone in the lateral head of the gastrocnemius) a loose body.

SEVERE COMMINUTED FRACTURES

These should be treated by internal fixation, if possible, either with screws, Kirschner wires, blade plates or Rush nails; alternatively by early movement and non-weight bearing on crutches.

KNEE INJURIES

DISLOCATION OF KNEE

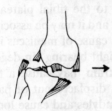

Examine for Damage to
Popliteal Vessels & Nerves

Aspirate Haemarthrosis

Reduce Dislocation

Repair Ligaments if Necessary

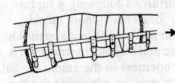

Wool + Pressure Bandage

Thomas Splint 3 Days

THEN   Cylinder Plaster
        for 6 Weeks

SEVERELY COMMINUTED FRACTURES

INTERNAL FIXATION

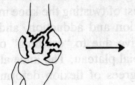

Examine for Vascular
and Neurological Damage

Aspirate Haemarthrosis

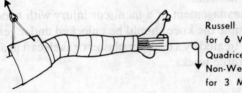

Russell Traction
for 6 Weeks

Quadriceps Exercises

Non-Weight-Bearing
for 3 Months

MENISCUS INJURIES

The medial meniscus is torn in about two-thirds of cases because of its firmer attachment to the tibial plateau and its attachment to the medial ligament and it may be associated with tears of the medial ligament. The cause of meniscus injuries is usually a twisting strain while weight bearing. In degenerative menisci, however, any type of strain may cause a tear. The bucket handle tear may result in displacement of part of the meniscus between the femoral condyles and cause locking.

The synovial effusion in a meniscus tear may take several hours to form while a haemarthrosis following a rupture of a medial ligament or a fracture forms much more quickly.

A diagnosis of a meniscus tear may also be made on the history of recurrent locking of the knee and inability to straighten it. On examination there is often tenderness in the antero-medial or antero-lateral joint lines, with pain on **adducting** the knee in medial meniscus tears and abducting the knee in lateral meniscus tears. With medial or lateral ligament injuries the reverse is true. In addition, the McMurray test of twisting the knee into various degrees of flexion in abduction and adduction, and trying to obtain a click, may be positive due to "catching" of the torn meniscus between the the tibial plateau. The knee also may be locked with about 10-20 degrees of flexion deformity with a "spongy" feel on attempted extension. A marked effusion into the knee may also prevent full extension, and this may make diagnosis more difficult.

If operative management of a meniscus injury with a locked knee is not possible the knee should be unlocked under general anaesthetic and treated by a cylinder plaster or skelecast in about 20° flexion for three weeks.

MENISCUS INJURIES OF THE KNEE

60% MEDIAL MENISCUS

 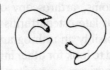 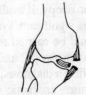

| BUCKET HANDLE | ANTERIOR OR POSTERIOR TAGS | ASSOCIATED WITH MEDIAL LIGAMENT RUPTURE |

CAUSATION

Weight Bearing
+
Twisting Strain

DIAGNOSIS

(Meniscus Injury Alone)

Synovial Effusion

Inability to Straighten

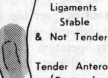

Ligaments Stable & Not Tender

Tender Antero (Postero) Medial Joint Line

TREATMENT

Meniscus Injury Alone

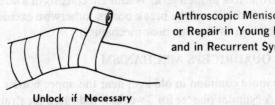

Arthroscopic Meniscectomy or Repair in Young Patients and in Recurrent Symptoms

Unlock if Necessary
Crepe Bandage

ENERGETIC QUADRICEPS EXERCISES FOR SEVERAL MONTHS

In young patients where the patient requires to return to early activity, such as in the case of a professional footballer, immediate meniscectomy or repair of a peripheral tear is indicated by arthroscopy, if available. In other cases, if the knee locks again or gives significant symptoms, arthroscopy or open meniscectomy should be carried out as late osteoarthritis may occur.

Arthroscopy, and possibly an arthrogram, may be indicated to confirm a diagnosis, and to look for other injuries. All knee injuries require energetic quadriceps exercises immediately, and a supporting bandage if a cylinder support is not used. In anterior cruciate tears, hamstring exercises are also indicated.

EXTENSOR MECHANISM OF KNEE

LIGAMENTUM PATELLAE AND ITS INSERTION

This is an injury common to the adolescent and young adults, caused by over use in jumpers and soccer players. Ice and physiotherapy are required for strains while ruptures require **early** operation.

In adolescent boys, an osteochondritis of the insertion of the ligamentum patellae is called Osgood-Schlatters disease. This requires rest and may need a protective back slab in severe cases.

SEPARATION OF THE PATELLA

This commonly occurs in middle age with the patella being pulled in two due to a sudden jerk. Treatment consists of a screw or tension band wire if a clean break occurs, otherwise excision and reconstruction of the extensor mechanism.

TEARS OF QUADRICEPS MECHANISM

These are more common in old age, near the upper border of the patella. A cylinder plaster for 3 weeks is indicated for strains and partial ruptures, and operation for complete rupture after haemarthrosis aspiration.

KNEE INJURIES

DAMAGE TO EXTENSOR MECHANISM

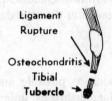

Ligament
Rupture

Osteochondritis

Tibial
Tubercle

LIGAMENTUM PATELLAE
(Young Patients)

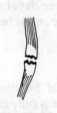

FRACTURE
PATELLA
(Middle Age)

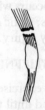

EXTENSOR
INSERTION
(Old Patients)

DIAGNOSIS

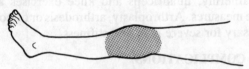

Haemarthrosis

Inability to Hold Up Leg Against Gravity

TREATMENT

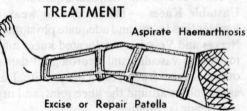

Repair
Complete
Rupture
Ligament
or
Extensor
Mechanism

Aspirate Haemarthrosis

Excise or Repair Patella
(See Fractures of the Patella)
SKELECAST IDEAL

ENERGETIC < EARLY STATIC
LATE ACTIVE > QUADRICEPS EXERCISES

COMPLICATIONS OF KNEE INJURIES

QUADRICEPS WASTING

This occurs within three days in all knee injuries. Quadriceps exercises, static or active, must be started **not** later than the day after any injury.

KNEE STIFFNESS

Knee exercises should be started as soon as possible and continued until the knee is fully mobile. Haemarthroses, unless minimal, should **always** be aspirated under full sterile precautions.

LATE OSTEOARTHRITIS

This is common if the joint surfaces are left irregular, if the knee is left in varus or valgus, or if loose bodies are present. Short wave diathermy, quadriceps and knee exercises are useful palliative measures. Arthroplasty, arthrodesis or osteotomy may be necessary for severe pain and stiffness.

OTHER COMPLICATIONS

(1) **Locking, Clicking and Giving Way** —These may be caused by loose bodies and meniscal injuries.
(2) **Unstable Knees** —This is due to weak quadriceps and ligamentous laxity, and adequate physiotherapy is essential.
(3) **Nerves and Vessels** —Dislocated knees may be responsible for severe vascular and neurological damage, as may any other severe fractures. The popliteal artery has poor anastomoses around the knee joint, and urgent exploration and repair is essential.

Microsurgical techniques should be used for nerve repair, but these are best delayed for **at least** 3 weeks in all severe knee injuries, both to allow the remainder of the knee to settle, as well as to localise the extent of fibrosis in the nerve following damage. This is discussed under nerve injuries.

KNEE INJURIES
COMPLICATIONS

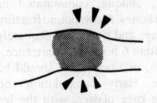 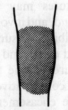

STIFFNESS AND PAIN | **RECURRENT EFFUSION**

 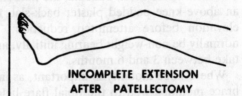

CHONDROMALACIA PATELLAE | **INCOMPLETE EXTENSION AFTER PATELLECTOMY**

 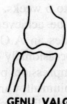 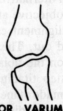

DAMAGE TO POPLITEAL ARTERY AND NERVES | **GENU VALGUM OR VARUM**

WEAKNESS AND GIVING WAY | **OSTEOARTHRITIS, LOOSE BODIES AND LOCKING**

FRACTURES OF THE SHAFT OF THE TIBIA AND FIBULA

Fractures may be transverse, oblique, comminuted or compound, and involve one or both bones. A compound fracture of the tibia is a surgical emergency, and must be adequately debrided early, and in any case within 6 hours of occurrence.

Fractures of the tibia and fibula, or tibia alone, should be treated conservatively if possible. Early manipulation and complete encasement in an above-knee plaster, with the leg elevated, is the treatment of choice. After manipulation the knee should be in about 10°-20° of flexion.

If there is too much oedema, the tibia should be treated with an above-knee padded plaster back-slab for a few days, plus elevation before attempted reduction. The patient should normally be non-weight bearing initially, and union will usually take between 3 and 6 months.

Where knee mobility is important, as in old patients, a cast brace moulded well to the tibial flare below the knee, with a padding over the ligamentum patellae, may allow mobility of the knee. Alternatively a skelecast with a knee hinge will achieve the same objective after 3 to 6 weeks.

If alignment cannot be achieved internal fixation must be carried out. This includes an A.O. or Huckstep compression plate on the tibia, or occasionally an intramedullary nail. The Huckstep titanium compression plate has the advantages of being made of inert titanium alloy and having grooves on its tibial surface to diminish the likelihood of periosteal vascular compression.

In a compound fracture, after adequate debridement, the skin should be left open if the wound is dirty. In the case of compound wounds, after adequate debridement, fixation can be achieved with 2 or 3 pins above and below the cortices of the tibia and held with compression on one or both sides. This is particularly valuable in compound fractures with vascular or neurological damage and is called an external fixateur.

FRACTURES OF TIBIA and FIBULA (SHAFT)

OBLIQUE
Twisting Force

TRANSVERSE
Lateral Force

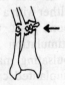

COMPOUND
Often Comminuted and
due to Direct Violence

INITIAL TREATMENT

Admit to Hospital
Elevate Limb

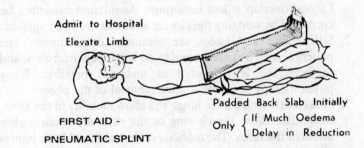

**FIRST AID -
PNEUMATIC SPLINT**

Padded Back Slab Initially

Only { If Much Oedema
Delay in Reduction

REDUCTION

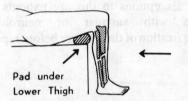

Pad under
Lower Thigh

Surgeon Seated and Fracture
Reduced
Below-Knee Plaster Applied
Before Extending it ABOVE
the Knee

In clean compound fractures intramedullary fixation with a nail is occasionally indicated in skilled hands.

Unstable oblique fractures can be held with a Steinmann's pin in the lower tibia with traction of 4 to 5 kgs.

In established non-union compression fixation should be either with a compression plate or with external compressors and bone graft. Good results can also be obtained with electrical stimulation with either an implanted battery, an external pulsating magnetic field, or ideally an external battery and implanted cathode leads in the form of insulated Kirschner wires. Twenty microamps of negative current given by each of 4 leads is ideal as a stimulus to new bone formation and the union of difficult fractures.

ADDITIONAL POINTS AND TREATMENT

1. Correction of angulation and shortening are important. Lateral overlap is less important. Angulation can often be corrected by wedging the plaster after this has been applied.
2. Stiff ankles and knees are common complications. The patient should be encouraged to do quadriceps exercises, and to keep the leg elevated as much as possible. Early physiotherapy is essential after removal of the plaster.
3. A skelecast with a knee hinge will allow mobility of the knee. Skelecasts allow for viewing of the skin and often earlier union of fractures. The mobility of the ankle and knee joint is also regained much more quickly than in a plaster support.
4. Internal fixation is indicated where adequate reduction cannot be obtained, or where early mobility is important. It should normally be confined to those patients who have no damage to the skin. Exceptions to this are patients with compound fractures with vascular or neurological complications needing fixation of the fracture before repair to the nerve or vessels.

FRACTURES OF TIBIA and FIBULA (SHAFT)

POST REDUCTION

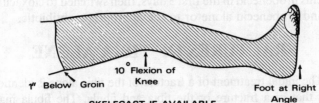

1" Below Groin

10° Flexion of Knee

Foot at Right Angle

SKELECAST IF AVAILABLE

Complete   Padded   Above - Knee   Plaster
3 months approx. Elevate until Oedema Settled
Non - Weight - Bearing   with   Crutches   Initially

AFTER UNION OF FRACTURE

| Energetic Knee and Ankle Exercises | Crepe Bandage or Elastoplast | Elevation of Leg when Sitting |

OTHER METHODS OF TREATMENT

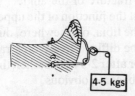

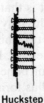

4-5 kgs

OBLIQUE FRACTURES WITH UNREDUCED SHORTENING

Steinmann's Pin through Lower Tibia

Huckstop Titanium Compression Plate

Intramedullary Nail and Huckstep Circlip

INTERNAL FIXATION

COMPRESSION PLATE WHERE POSSIBLE

5. In compound fractures, in addition to extensive debridement and drainage, the patient must be given prophylactic tetanus toxoid or tetanus immunoglobulin, as well as a wide spectrum of antibiotics such as cloxacillin, ampicillin and penicillin, plus probenecid in the first 3 days, then switched to cloxacillin and probenecid alone or to the appropriate antibiotic.

FRACTURES OF TIBIA ALONE

The initial treatment of a fracture of the tibia alone is identical with that of a fracture of the tibia and fibula. The fibula may, however, act as a strut and prevent union of the tibia by holding the two fracture ends apart. If non-union appears to be occurring, a small segment (about 2cm) of the fibula should be excised through a lateral incision so as to allow the ends of the tibia to come together or the fibula cut obliquely to allow overlap.

OTHER FRACTURES OF THE TIBIA

These can be classified as follows:

1. **Associated with a Fracture of the Ankle Joint** — The ankle must always be examined in all fractures of the tibia and fibula. Management is that of the fracture of the ankle.

2. **Stress Fracture** — This may occur at the junction of the upper one-third and lower two-thirds of the tibia, or elsewhere, due to unaccustomed exercise. It may be difficult to see on x-ray and only diagnosed on bone scan, or after 2-3 weeks when the fracture site and callus formation become obvious.

COMPOUND AND COMMINUTED FRACTURES OF TIBIA

External Fixation (Single)   External Fixation (Double)

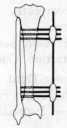 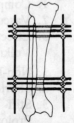

With Methyl Methacrylate
Cement or Fixateurs

Compression plus
Adjustment with Fixateurs

FRACTURES OF FIBULA ALONE

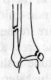

ASSOCIATED WITH
ANKLE FRACTURES

STRESS
FRACTURE

ALL OTHER
FRACTURES

↓

TREAT AS FOR
ANKLE FRACTURES

Crepe Bandage
OR
Below-Knee Walking
Plaster or Strapping
for 3 Weeks
Then
Crepe Bandage and
Ankle Exercises

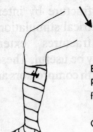

COMPLICATIONS OF FRACTURES OF THE SHAFT OF THE TIBIA AND THE FIBULA

EARLY
1. Compound Fracture — Osteomyelitis.
2. Vascular Damage — Gangrene.
3. Effects of Tight Plasters — Pressure Sores, Volkmann's Ischaemic Contracture, Gangrene

LATE
1. Non-Union — Especially Lower Third.
2. Shortening — Especially with Oblique Fractures.
3. Stiff Ankle and Knee — Especially with Prolonged Immobilisation

NON-UNION OF THE TIBIA & FIBULA

Non-union of the tibia is common at the junction of the upper two-thirds and lower one-third due to the poor blood supply at the site. Infection and faulty immobilisation of the fracture site are other important causes. Established non-union usually requires operation. The bone ends may require freshening and a compression plate. Bone chips from the iliac crest are used to bridge the fracture site. Other methods include a sliding bone graft from the shaft of the tibia, and a Huckstep 10.5 mm compression nail or Huckstep grooved titanium compression plate. The electrical bone stimulator may also be indicated. Stabilisation of the fracture by internal or external means is important when electrical stimulation is used.

In compound fractures external compression with compression pins may be useful. These are applied either on one side of the tibia, or with compressors and pins on both sides of the tibia as illustrated.

COMPLICATIONS OF FRACTURES OF TIBIA and FIBULA

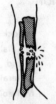

COMPOUND FRACTURE

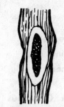

OSTEOMYELITIS following **COMPOUND FRACTURE**

ARTERY OR NERVE DAMAGE Usually Following Compound Fracture

NON-UNION Lower 1/3 i.e. Poor Blood Supply

SHORTENING Oblique Fractures

MALUNION Late Osteoarthritis of Ankle

STIFFNESS OF KNEE Inadequate Physiotherapy

STIFFNESS AND OEDEMA OF ANKLE Inadequate Physiotherapy

PRESSURE SORES UNDER PLASTER Badly Applied or Unpadded Plaster

LIGAMENTOUS INJURIES OF THE ANKLE

CAUSATION   EXAMINATION

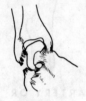

Tender and
Swelling over
Ligament

Check Calcaneus
Talus and
Talo-Calcaneal
Ligaments

Forced Inversion

Check
Medial
and
Lateral
Malleoli

Check Base
5th Metatarsal

X-RAY FOR COMPLICATIONS

Rupture
Inferior Tibio-Fibular
Ligament with Diastasis

Fracture

ANKLE   TALUS

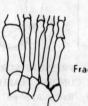

Fracture

Fracture

5th METATARSAL   CALCANEUS

LIGAMENTOUS INJURIES

TREATMENT

SPRAIN

PARTIAL RUPTURE

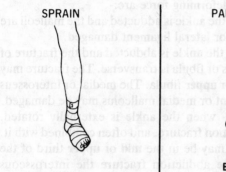

Crepe Bandage Over Wool

Below-Knee Walking
Plaster 3 - 6 Weeks

COMPLETE RUPTURE

EARLY TREATMENT

UNTREATED LATE
RUPTURES

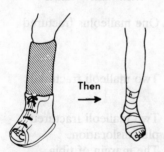

Then →

Below-Knee Plaster   Crepe Bandage
and Overboot
SKELECAST
WHERE POSSIBLE

Outside Wedge
in Heel +

  Or

FRACTURES OF THE ANKLE

DEFORMING FORCE

· The three types of deforming force are:-

1. **Adduction** — when the ankle is adducted and the malleoli are displaced medially or lateral ligament damaged.
2. **Abduction** — when the ankle is abducted and the fracture of the lateral malleolus or fibula is transverse. The fracture may also be in the **mid** or **upper** fibula. The medial or interosseus tibio-fibular ligament or medial malleolus may be damaged.
3. **External Rotation** - when the ankle is externally rotated. Similar to an abduction fracture, and often combined with it. Again the fracture may be in the **mid** or **upper** third of the fibula. As with the abduction fracture the interosseous tibio-fibular and medial ligaments may be ruptured and require operation and also the medial malleolus fractured.

CLASSIFICATION — COMMON FRACTURES

A useful classification of ankle fractures is as follows:

1°
1. Adduction
2. Abduction
3. External rotation
} One malleolus fractured

2°
1. Adduction
2. Abduction
3. External rotation
} Two malleoli fractured

3°
1. Adduction
2. Abduction
3. External rotation
} Two malleoli fractured plus dislocation. The margin of tibia may be fractured and tibio-fibular and medial ligaments ruptured.

FRACTURES OF THE ANKLE
FIRST DEGREE
(One Malleolus)

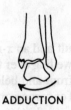
ADDUCTION

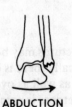
ABDUCTION

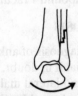
EXTERNAL ROTATION

TREATMENT

Most Cases   **OR**

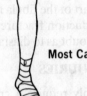

Crepe Bandage + Crutches
+ Early Weight Bearing

Displaced Fracture
Medial Malleolus

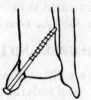

Internal Fixation

FURTHER TREATMENT

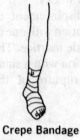

Crepe Bandage

PLUS

Energetic Ankle
and Foot
Exercises

Ⓟ

CLASSIFICATION — UNCOMMON FRACTURES

(1) Transverse force
(2) Vertical force
(3) Compound Fracture

DIAGNOSIS

The diagnosis of ankle fractures may be difficult, and an x-ray is essential if in doubt. Clinically there is often swelling over the medial and lateral malleoli, as well as over the front and below the malleoli, and local tenderness is common. Tenderness may also occur in these areas with severe sprains of the lateral ligament of the ankle.

The talus, calcaneus and base of the 5th metatarsal should also be examined. The 5th metatarsal base may be pulled off by the peroneus brevis tendon. The mid or upper part of the fibula may also be fractured in external rotation or abduction fractures of the ankle. Oblique x-rays are essential if in doubt as to diastasis.

FIRST DEGREE AND LIGAMENTOUS INJURIES

These usually need no reduction and only require a crepe bandage, wool and crutches for 3 days. Gradually increasing full weight bearing can then be started in most cases. Sometimes a walking plaster or a skelecast may be required for 3 weeks. In **complete** tears of the lateral and medial ligaments, immobilisation may have to be continued for 6 weeks.

Fractures of the medial malleolus, with displacement or rotation, may require accurate reduction and fixation with one or two screws as it is essential to have a perfect ankle mortice. The lateral malleolus may also require internal fixation with a small plate if displaced upwards with associated rupture of the interosseous tibio-fibular ligament.

FRACTURES OF THE ANKLE
SECOND DEGREE
(Two Malleoli)

 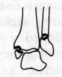

ADDUCTION   **ABDUCTION**   **EXTERNAL ROTATION**

TREATMENT

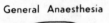

General Anaesthesia

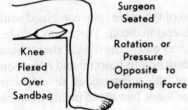 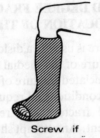

Knee Flexed Over Sandbag

Surgeon Seated

Rotation or Pressure Opposite to Deforming Force

Screw if Not Perfect Reduction

FURTHER TREATMENT

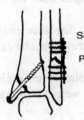

Screw + Plate

Plus

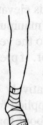

Crepe Bandage

SECOND DEGREE FRACTURES OF THE ANKLE

These may require reduction with or without internal fixation. Manipulation should be tried initially, except in cases where there is displacement of the medial malleolus in the top of the mortice, when accurate reduction is essential. After reduction a below-knee, non-weight bearing skelecast or plaster will be necessary for 3 to 6 weeks, followed by weight bearing. In severe fractures the immobilisation time may extend from 9 to 12 weeks. Where accurate reduction of the ankle cannot be obtained, screw fixation of the medial malleolus following plate, screw or Rush nail fixation of the lateral malleolus is essential, especially with lower tibio-fibular ligament rupture and diastasis.

THIRD DEGREE FRACTURE
DISLOCATION OF THE ANKLE

There is usually a dislocation of the ankle joint combined with a fracture of the medial and lateral malleoli. There may also be an associated fracture of the lower end of the tibia. Patients with these conditions all require admission to hospital and reduction of the fracture and repair of the interosseous tibio-fibular ligament. An attempt should be made initially to manipulate the ankle under general anaesthetic, **except** in severe cases where accurate reduction can only be obtained by open reduction.

If oedema is severe a below-knee padded back slab is given and the leg is elevated with crepe bandage and wool for 3 or 4 days **before** manipulation or operation.

Damage to the vessels or nerves due to the displacement must be looked for. If present an immediate reduction must be carried out.

Post-operatively a non-weight bearing plaster or skelecast should be applied for 6 weeks, followed by weight bearing in a canvas overboot for a further 3 to 6 weeks.

FRACTURES OF THE ANKLE
THIRD DEGREE
Fracture–Dislocation

ADDUCTION
Associated Fracture

ABDUCTION
Articular Surface

EXTERNAL ROTATION
Tibia Common

TREATMENT

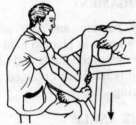

Manipulation
and Below-Knee
Padded Plaster

OR

Screw if Not
Perfect Reduction

Above-Knee in Very Unstable Fractures

FURTHER TREATMENT

Non-Weight-
Bearing Plaster

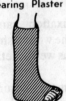

Weight-Bearing
Only after
6–9 Weeks

Crepe Bandage

Screw in
Failed Closed
Reduction

TOTAL TIME IN PLASTER 9–12 WEEKS

TREATMENT OF UNCOMMON FRACTURES OF THE ANKLE

VERTICAL FORCE

Treat with a below-knee non-weight bearing plaster or skelecast for 2 to 3 months and occasionally by internal fixation. Associated crush fractures of the calcaneus or lumbar spine should be looked for.

TRANSVERSE FORCE FRACTURES

The transverse force fracture is due to a sideways blow. It is usually impossible to hold accurately by closed manipulation, and both malleoli should usually be internally fixed.

RUPTURE OF TIBIO-FIBULAR LIGAMENT

The tibio-fibular ligament may rupture and the ankle displaced laterally. Treatment is by a screw or plate to hold the lateral malleolus. A screw, if used between the fibula and tibia, should be removed as soon as stability has been obtained and **before** unsupported full weight bearing.

COMPOUND FRACTURES OF THE ANKLE

A compound fracture of the ankle is treated in exactly the same way as a simple fracture. The patient must, however, be admitted to hospital and the leg elevated. The fracture must be reduced and adequate debridement of the wound carried out as an emergency **within** 6 hours of injury.

In clean compound fractures internal fixation can be attempted as with closed fractures. In **all** cases the wound should be drained and adequate chemotherapy given, as well as tetanus toxoid or tetanus immunoglobulin.

In the case of dirty wounds delayed primary closure is indicated. Chemotherapy should be continued for at least 3 weeks post-operatively and the leg kept elevated. Further treatment includes protection of the ankle by a skelecast, wool and a crepe bandage, and elevation to prevent oedema.

FRACTURES OF THE ANKLE

VERTICAL FORCE

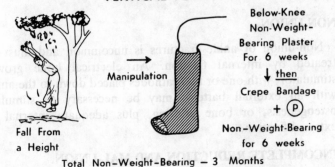

Fall From
a Height

Manipulation →

Below-Knee
Non-Weight-
Bearing Plaster
For 6 weeks
↓ then
Crepe Bandage
+ Ⓟ
Non-Weight-Bearing
for 6 weeks

Total Non-Weight-Bearing — 3 Months

TRANSVERSE FORCE

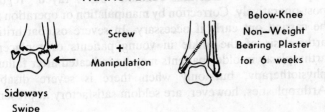

Sideways
Swipe

Screw
+
Manipulation
→

Below-Knee
Non-Weight
Bearing Plaster
for 6 weeks

RUPTURE TIBIO-FIBULAR LIGAMENT

Abduction or
External Rotation

→   Manipulation   OR   Screw

COMPLICATIONS OF FRACTURES OF THE ANKLE

NON-UNION

Non-union of ankle fractures is uncommon and must be treated by internal fixation. An electrical bone growth stimulator, with one or two cathodes placed down to the ankle with an external battery, may be necessary to stimulate osteogenesis, or bone grafting, plus adequate internal or external fixation.

INCOMPLETE REDUCTION AND MAL-UNION.

This is common and may lead to severe osteoarthritis. It is important that fractures should be x-rayed regularly post-operatively. Correction by manipulation or operation must be carried out early if necessary. In severe osteoarthritis an arthrodesis of the ankle in young patients or replacement arthroplasty in older patients may be indicated after failure of physiotherapy, but only when there is severe disability. Arthroplasties, however, are seldom satisfactory at present.

STIFFNESS AND PAIN

These are usually due to inadequate ankle exercises after removal of the plaster. They may also be due to inadequate reduction or osteoarthritis. Treatment should be by intensive physiotherapy and possibly manipulation under general anaesthetic.

OEDEMA

This is usually due to inadequate elevation and lack of ankle exercises. Treatment should be by elevation, wool, a crepe bandage, ankle support or elastic stocking plus adequate physiotherapy. Occasionally infection in a compound fracture will need chemotherapy.

INJURIES OF THE ANKLE
COMPLICATIONS

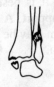

Non Union

Incomplete Reduction

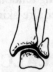

Osteoarthritis

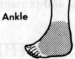

Ankle   Subtalar Joints

Stiffness, Oedema and Pain

Instability

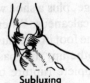

Subluxing Peroneal Tendons

Inability to Rise Up On Toe (Tendo Achillis Rupture)

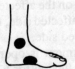

Pressure by Tight Plaster - Sores or Volkmann's Ischaemia

INSTABILITY

Instability of the ankle is usually due to inadequate physiotherapy after removal of the plaster. Occasionally it is due to the rupture of the lateral ligaments. It is best treated by adequate physiotherapy plus an elastic support. A raise on the outer side of the sole of the shoe of 0.5 cm may be indicated to diminish the likelihood of ankle inversion.

OTHER COMPLICATIONS

These include subluxing peroneal tendons, and pressure by a tight incompletely padded plaster. Subluxing tendons may need to be stabilised and pressure sores may require skin grafting.

INJURIES TO THE TENDO CALCANEUS

These are often due to unaccustomed running or sport in middle age. A strain or partial rupture is treated by a supporting bandage, plus a shoe with an extra heel to take the strain off the tendo calcaneus. Where the pain is severe a plaster or skelecast with the foot in equinus is required for about 3 weeks followed by physiotherapy and passive stretching to regain dorsiflexion.

Complete rupture of the tendo calcaneus causes a gap with weakness of plantar flexion of the ankle. The long flexors of the toe and the tendon of plantaris may be able to plantarflex the foot weakly, but the patient will **not** usually be able to rise up on his toes on the affected side. In addition, when squeezing the calf on the affected side, the foot will **not** plantarflex, as it will on the uninjured side.

Treatment is operative repair followed by the foot held in plantar flexion for 6 weeks in a plaster or skelecast. Operative repair leads to better results than conservative management alone. Physiotherapy is necessary to regain dorsiflexion after repair.

INJURY TO TENDO CALCANEUS

STRAIN
TREATMENT

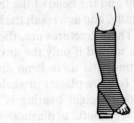

Shoe with
Extra Heel
+
Strapping

OR

Plaster with
Foot in Equinus

COMPLETE RUPTURE

EXAMINATION	TREATMENT

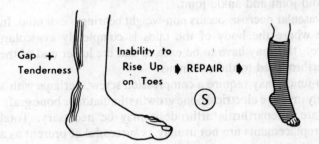

Gap +
Tenderness

Inability to
Rise Up ▸ REPAIR ▸
on Toes
Ⓢ

Ability to Plantarflex
Foot with Long Flexors
of Toes

Plaster in Full Equinus
6 Weeks
Non-Weight-Bearing

MAJOR FRACTURES OF THE TALUS

Major fractures are those involving the neck of the talus, with or without displacement. The blood supply to the talus, as with the scaphoid and the head of the femur, comes mainly from the capsule distally, and as a result the blood supply to the body may be cut off. These fractures are, therefore, surgical emergencies and may be missed if only the ankle joint is seen on x-ray.

The treatment, if there is no displacement, is a below-knee non-weight bearing plaster or skelecast for 2 to 3 months. It is **important** that weight bearing is **not** started too soon. Bone scanning is very useful to diagnose whether the blood supply has been cut off and the body of the talus is viable.

In cases where there is displacement, reduction by manipulation may be necessary with internal fixation with one or two compression screws or Kirschner wires.

COMPLICATIONS

Complications of fractures of the talus include avascular necrosis of the body, non-union and late osteoarthritis of the subtaloid joint and ankle joint.

If avascular necrosis occurs non-weight bearing is essential. In a case where the body of the talus is completely avascular, however, this may have to be excised and the lower end of the tibia arthrodesed to the calcaneus.

Non-union may require a compression screw, perhaps with a partially invasive electrical bone growth stimulator or bone graft.

In late osteoarthritis arthrodesis may be necessary. Total ankle replacements are not usually as successful at present as a good arthrodesis.

FRACTURES OF THE TALUS

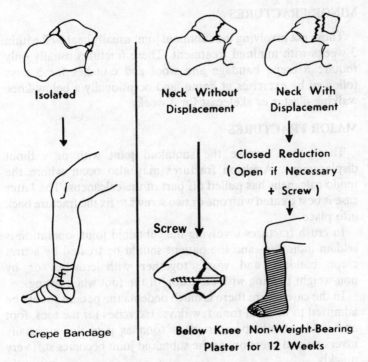

Isolated

Neck Without Displacement

Neck With Displacement

↓

**Closed Reduction
(Open if Necessary
+ Screw)**

Screw

Crepe Bandage

**Below Knee Non-Weight-Bearing
Plaster for 12 Weeks**

COMPLICATIONS
(Fracture Neck of Talus)

Avascular Necrosis

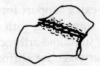

Subtaloid Osteoarthritis

FRACTURES OF THE CALCANEUS

MINOR FRACTURES

Those **not** involving the subtaloid joint usually heal well within 3 weeks with minimal treatment. These fractures usually only require a crepe bandage and wool and crutches for 3 days followed by exercises at home, and occasionally a below-knee walking plaster or skelecast for 3 weeks.

MAJOR FRACTURES

These may involve the subtaloid joint with or without displacement. Avulsion fractures may also occur where the tendo calcaneus has pulled off part of the calcaneus. The latter case is best treated with one or two screws to fix the fracture back into place.

In crush fractures involving the subtaloid joint, operation is **seldom** indicated, and the patient should be treated by a firm crepe bandage and wool, together with crutches or by non-weight bearing with elevation of the foot when sitting.

In the case where there is much oedema the patient should be admitted to hospital for a few days. Exercises for the toes, foot and ankle should be started as soon as possible, especially inversion and eversion, as the subtaloid joint becomes stiff very quickly.

The patient should be **non**-weight bearing for at least 6 weeks and sometimes two or three months, as too early weight bearing will crush the calcaneus further and lead to osteoarthritis and pain. There is an occasional place for a below the knee plaster to give extra support for 3 to 6 weeks.

In some cases with severe crushing there may be a place for early subtaloid arthrodesis. This may in any case be necessary at a later stage for stiffness and pain.

FRACTURES OF THE CALCANEUS

  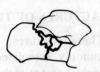

**NOT Involving
Joint**

**Subtalar Joint
Without Displacement**

**Subtalar Joint
With Displacement**

CAUSES

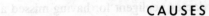

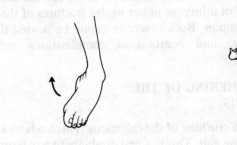 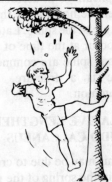

TWIST

FALL FROM A HEIGHT

TREATMENT
(FRACTURE NOT INVOLVING
SUBTALAR JOINT)

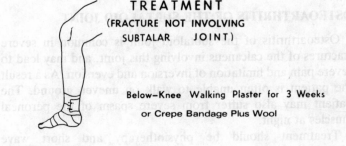

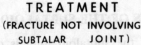

**Below–Knee Walking Plaster for 3 Weeks
or Crepe Bandage Plus Wool**

COMPLICATIONS OF FRACTURES OF THE CALCANEUS

FRACTURES OF THE SPINE

These fractures, particularly in the lumbar region, are commonly associated with fractures of the calcaneus. It is therefore essential that in all calcaneal fractures a lateral x- ray of the lumbar spine be carried out, **even though** the patient does not complain of back pain. This is because there are often legal complications in accidents, and the patient may later consider either the hospital or the doctor negligent for having missed a fracture of the spine. Later it will be difficult to prove that this did not occur at the time of injury, as minor wedge fractures of the lumbar spine are common. Back exercises should be started if there is a fracture, and neurological complications are uncommon.

RELATIVE LENGTHENING OF THE TENDO CALCANEUS

This may be due to crushing of the calcaneus. This leads to a loss in the spring of the gait. This is a real disability to a patient who has to climb ladders, particularly as fractures of the calcaneus are common in window cleaners and builders.

OSTEOARTHRITIS OF THE SUBTALOID JOINT

Osteoarthritis of the subtaloid joint is common in severe fractures of the calcaneus involving this joint, and may lead to severe pain and limitation of inversion and eversion. As a result the patient is often unable to walk on uneven ground. The patient may also suffer from severe spasm of the peroneal muscles at night.

Treatment should be physiotherapy and short wave diathermy. In severe disability arthrodesis of the subtaloid joint may be necessary. In very severe crush fractures there may be a place for immediate subtaloid arthrodesis

FRACTURES OF THE CALCANEUS

TREATMENT

(FRACTURES INVOLVING SUBTALAR JOINT)

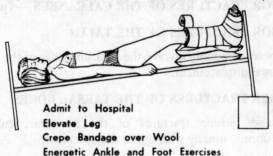

Admit to Hospital
Elevate Leg
Crepe Bandage over Wool
Energetic Ankle and Foot Exercises.

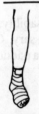

Energetic Ankle and Foot Exercises
Inversion and Eversion
Particularly

Most Cases	**Occasionally**
Crepe Bandage and	Below Knee.
Non-Weight-Bearing	Non-Weight-Bearing
for 2 Months from Fracture	Plaster for 3 - 6 Weeks

COMPLICATIONS

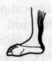

Crush Fracture		**Osteoarthritis**
Vertebrae (Also	**Relative Lengthening**	**Pain and**
Fracture Base Skull)	**Tendo Calcaneus**	**Stiffness**

MINOR FRACTURES OF THE TARSAL BONES

MINOR FRACTURES OF THE CALCANEUS — (page 354.)

MINOR FRACTURES OF THE TALUS

These commonly involve the back and sides of the talus with minimal displacement.

OTHER FRACTURES OF THE TARSAL BONES

These include fractures of the navicular, cuboid and cuneiforms, usually with minor displacement.

TREATMENT

These all heal well with little residual disability. A crepe bandage for 3 weeks is usually all that is necessary. Graduated weight bearing is possible. Only occasionally is a padded walking plaster for 3 weeks necessary.

COMPLICATIONS

Pain, stiffness and osteoarthritis of the joints involved may occasionally occur and require physiotherapy.

MID-TARSAL FRACTURE DISLOCATION

A mid-tarsal fracture dislocation, often with dislocation of the talus on the navicular and cuneiforms on the tarsus, frequently occurs in association with a fracture of the metatarsals and cuboid, and is a surgical emergency. Both the dorsalis pedis and tibialis posterior arteries may be compressed, with ischaemia of the toes. There is often diminution of sensation associated with a colder foot than on the opposite side.

FRACTURES OF THE TARSUS

(Excluding Talus and Calcaneus)

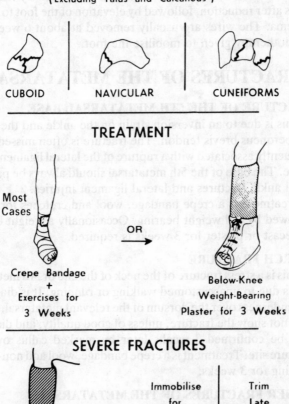

CUBOID · NAVICULAR · CUNEIFORMS

TREATMENT

Most Cases

Crepe Bandage
+
Exercises for
3 Weeks
Ⓟ

OR

Below-Knee
Weight-Bearing
Plaster for 3 Weeks

SEVERE FRACTURES

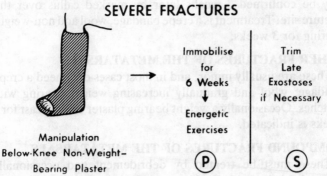

Manipulation
Below-Knee Non-Weight-
Bearing Plaster
Ⓟ

Immobilise
for
6 Weeks
+
Energetic
Exercises

Trim
Late
Exostoses
if Necessary
Ⓢ

It is important that this is treated as a **surgical emergency** and the patient **admitted** to hospital. The fracture is usually very unstable and best results are obtained by fixation by Kirschner wires after reduction, followed by elevation of the foot to reduce oedema. The wires are usually removed at about 6 weeks and physiotherapy given to mobilise the foot.

FRACTURES OF THE METATARSALS

FRACTURE OF THE 5TH METATARSAL BASE

This is due to an inversion strain on the ankle and the pull of the peroneus brevis tendon. The fracture is often missed and is frequently associated with a rupture of the lateral ligament of the ankle. The base of the 5th metatarsal should always be palpated in all ankle fractures and lateral ligament injuries.

Treatment is a crepe bandage, wool and crutches for 3 days followed by full weight bearing. Occasionally a weight bearing skelecast or plaster for 3 weeks is required.

MARCH FRACTURE

This is a stress fracture of the neck of the 2nd or 3rd metatarsal necks due to unaccustomed walking or running. It is diagnosed by tenderness over the dorsum of the relevant metatarsal. X-rays may not show the fracture, unless of good quality, and diagnosis may be confirmed 3 weeks later by marked callus over the fracture site. Treatment is a crepe bandage, wool and non-weight bearing for 3 weeks.

OTHER FRACTURES OF THE METATARSALS

These are usually minor, and in most cases only need a crepe bandage, wool and gradually increasing weight bearing with crutches. Occasionally a weight bearing plaster or skelecast for 3 weeks is indicated.

COMPOUND FRACTURES OF THE METATARSALS

These must be treated by debridement and occasionally internal fixation with Kirschner wires.

FRACTURES OF THE METATARSALS

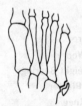

BASE 5TH

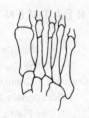

MARCH FRACTURE
FAINT CRACK
2ND OR 3RD NECK

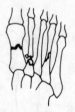

ALL OTHER
FRACTURES

CAUSES

INWARD
TWIST
OF FOOT
Peroneus
Brevis
Pulls Off
Insertion

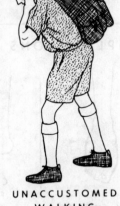

UNACCUSTOMED
WALKING
STRESS FRACTURE

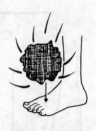

DIRECT TRAUMA
OR TWISTING
Transverse Oblique
or Comminuted
Often Multiple
Sometimes Compound

FRACTURES OF THE METATARSALS

TREATMENT

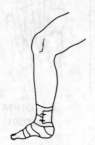

Most Only Require
Crepe Bandage + Wool
Crutches + Gradual Full Weight Bearing
Occasionally Walking Plaster
or Plastic Below Knee
Seldom Require Manipulation

FURTHER TREATMENT

Crepe Bandage or Strapping	Firm Soled Boot or Shoe	Foot and Ankle Exercises

COMPLICATIONS

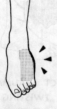

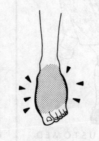

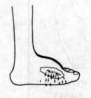

LOCALISED
TENDERNESS

PAIN SWELLING
AND STIFFNESS

COMPOUND
FRACTURE
and
OSTEOMYELITIS

FRACTURES OF THE TOES

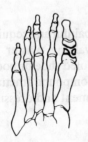 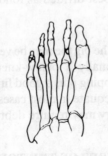 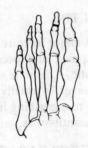

BIG TOE   **MULTIPLE FRACTURES**   **SINGLE FRACTURE**
                 2ND - 5TH TOES   **2ND - 5TH TOES**

CAUSES

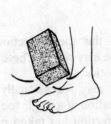 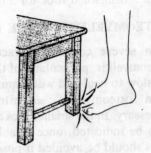

HEAVY WEIGHT   **KICKING AGAINST**
                         CHAIR OR STONE

FRACTURES OF THE TOES

Most fractures of the toes are minor but they can be very painful. They can be best divided as follows.

BIG TOE

A major fracture of the big toe may be very painful and require strapping and occasionally a below-knee walking plaster or plastic. Adequate strapping plus a good firm soled shoe or boot, however, is usually adequate in most cases. Compound fracture due to a crushing injury may require debridement and dressing plus antibiotics.

MULTIPLE FRACTURES OF THE TOES

These can be treated by strapping or occasionally in a below-knee walking plaster or skelecast for 3 weeks.

SINGLE FRACTURES OF THE OTHER TOES

A single fracture seldom requires to be reduced. It is best treated with strapping either by itself or to the adjoining toe for 3 weeks.

This fracture can be very painful and the patient is advised to wear a firm soled shoe for 3 or 4 weeks.

OSTEOMYELITIS OF THE TOES

In severe compound fractures of the toes infection or osteomyelitis, particularly of the big toe may result. These may be slow to heal and will require antibiotics.

In osteomyelitis sequestrectomy may occasionally be necessary. In the smaller toes an amputation of a single toe may also be indicated, once established infection has taken place. This should be avoided if possible in the big toe.

FRACTURES OF THE TOES

BIG TOE

SINGLE TOE

**MULTIPLE FRACTURES
AND OTHER TOES**

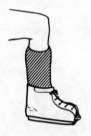

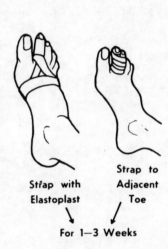

Below Knee Walking
Plaster for 3 Weeks
Reduction Rarely Necessary
Strapping May Be Adequate

Strap with
Elastoplast

Strap to
Adjacent
Toe

For 1—3 Weeks

COMPLICATIONS

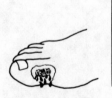

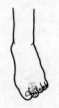

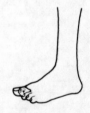

OSTEOMYELITIS

STIFFNESS
OEDEMA PAIN

DEFORMITY AND
PRESSURE ON SHOE

POST-OPERATIVE CARE

POST-OPERATIVE TREATMENT OF INJURIES

UPPER LIMB

1. Elevation of the limb either by a "roller towel" or on pillows for at least three days post-operatively. Outpatients should have the arm elevated in a sling. The patient should move the fingers, elbow and shoulder as much as possible.
2. Check the fingers regularly for appearance, warmth, movement, ability to straighten the fingers, swelling and sensation, **disturbing** the patient if necessary. The plaster should be checked for pressure.
3. If the circulation is in doubt, the plaster should be split or loosened **immediately.** In supracondylar fractures, the elbow should be extended. (See supracondylar fracture) and the patient treated as an emergency.

LOWER LIMB

1. Elevation of the limb in major cases, either by bed blocks, or pillows, for at least 1 to 3 days post-operatively. The patient should move the toes frequently.
2. In acute cases, plasters should be either well padded and split, or a plaster slab and bandage used instead of a complete plaster.
3. On the evening of operation, it is important to check swelling, colour, warmth, sensation and movement of toes, disturbing the patient if necessary. Plaster should be trimmed if rough areas are causing pressure.
4. If there is any doubt as to the circulation the plaster should be split and loosened down to the **skin** for its **whole length** and opened out.

POST-OPERATIVE CARE

OBSERVATION OF CIRCULATION and PATIENT

FINGERS
AND } 1/2 Hourly { Appearance, Warmth and Pulses
TOES } { Movement and Sensation
{ Swelling and Plaster Pressure

PATIENT'S
GENERAL } Careful Observation { Chest
CONDITION } { Abdomen
{ Shock and Haemorrhage

SPLIT PLASTER
(IF IN DOUBT)

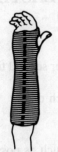

Split WHOLE Length
Down to SKIN itself
Open out WELL

Increase Elevation
Encourage Movement of
Fingers and Toes

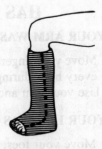

↓

AFTER SPLITTING PLASTER PUT WOOL
IN GAP AND CREPE BANDAGE

INSTRUCTIONS FOR PATIENTS IN PLASTER

IF YOUR ARM IS IN PLASTER

(1) Move your shoulder and fingers several times every hour during the day.
(2) Keep the plaster dry and away from water.
(3) Carry the arm in a sling during the first 3 days if your hand or fingers are at all swollen.

IF YOUR LEG IS IN PLASTER

(1) Do NOT bear weight on it UNLESS the plaster has a foot piece or you have been given an overboot.
(2) Move the toes several times every hour during the day.
(3) Raise your foot on a chair when sitting, especially during the first week.

If your fingers or toes become swollen or cannot be felt properly, go to the nearest hospital or inform your own doctor IMMEDIATELY.

INSTRUCTIONS AFTER THE PLASTER HAS BEEN REMOVED

IF YOUR ARM WAS INJURED

(1) Move your fingers, wrist, elbow and shoulder several times every hour during the day.
(2) Use your arm and hand more and more each day.

IF YOUR LEG WAS INJURED

(1) Move your toes, ankle, knee and hip as much as possible each day.
(2) If your foot swells, raise it on a stool when sitting, and wear a crepe bandage or elastic support, or stocking.
(3) Walk more and more each day.

INSTRUCTIONS TO PATIENTS
IN PLASTER

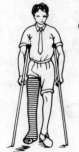

GOOD

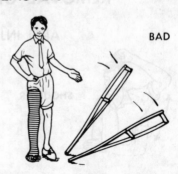

BAD

DO NOT BEAR WEIGHT ON PLASTER
Unless the Plaster has an Overboot or Footpiece

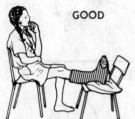

GOOD

BAD

ELEVATE ARM OR LEG WHEN SITTING
Move Fingers, Shoulder and Toes

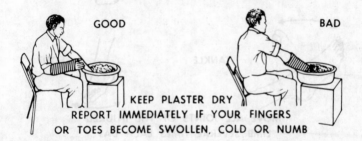

GOOD

BAD

KEEP PLASTER DRY
REPORT IMMEDIATELY IF YOUR FINGERS
OR TOES BECOME SWOLLEN, COLD OR NUMB

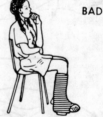

ADVICE TO PATIENTS AFTER REMOVAL OF PLASTER

ARM INJURIES

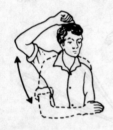

SHOULDER

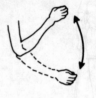

ELBOW

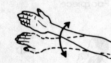

FOREARM

WRIST AND HAND

LEG INJURIES

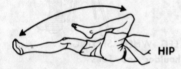

HIP

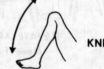

KNEE

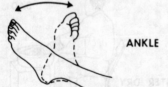

ANKLE

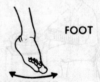

FOOT

MOVE ALL JOINTS OF THE INJURED LIMB SEVERAL TIMES EACH DAY

UPPER LIMB EXERCISES
ACTIVE AND PASSIVE

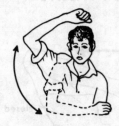

Abduction of Shoulder

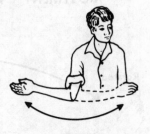

Internal and External
Rotation of Shoulder

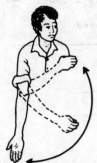

Flexion and Extension of
Elbow

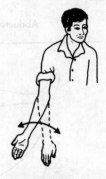

Pronation and Supination

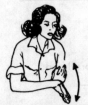

Flexion and Extension of
Wrist

Flexion and Extension of
Fingers

PREVENTION OF DEFORMITIES
MOVEMENT   ACTIVE OR PASSIVE

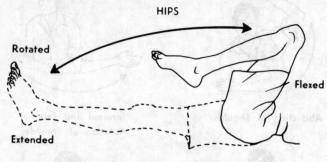

HIPS

Rotated

Flexed

Extended

Abducted and Adducted

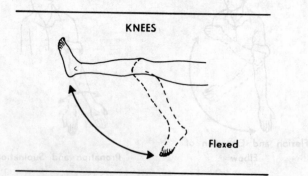

KNEES

Flexed

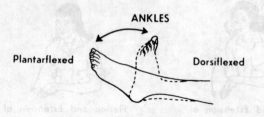

ANKLES

Plantarflexed   Dorsiflexed

Everted and Inverted

PHYSIOTHERAPY

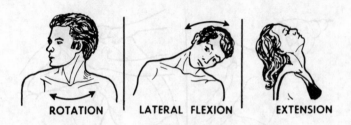

ROTATION   LATERAL FLEXION   EXTENSION

BACK EXERCISES

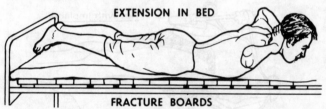

EXTENSION IN BED

FRACTURE BOARDS

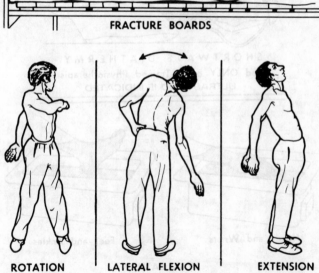

ROTATION   LATERAL FLEXION   EXTENSION

PHYSIOTHERAPY

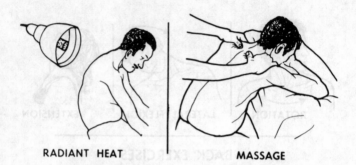

RADIANT HEAT

MASSAGE

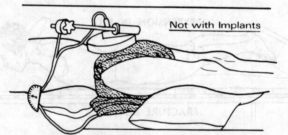

Not with Implants

SHORTWAVE DIATHERMY
Used ONLY by a Trained Physiotherapist
ULTRASOUND IF INDICATED

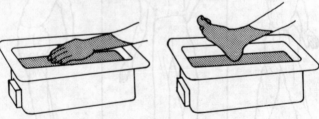

Hands and Wrists

Feet and Ankles

WAX BATHS

REHABILITATION

Adequate early physiotherapy will minimise late stiffness of joints and weakness of muscles, in nearly all injuries, and early rehabilitation is important in all severe trauma.

All patients with fractures and dislocations must be shown early movements of the relevant joints of the upper and lower limbs or back as illustrated.

After removal of plaster and skelecasts a crepe bandage and wool for a few days, with energetic exercises, either at home or in a physiotherapy department, is essential. The injured limb should also be elevated to prevent oedema. Swimming is particularly valuable for mobilising joints and strengthening muscles. Walking on soft sand in bare feet is good for ankle and joint injuries, while cycling on a static machine or actual bicycle is indicated for hip, knee and back injuries.

The long-term management of patients with amputations, residual paralysis, or residual deformities, requires a team approach with surgeons, physicians, social workers, or physiotherapists, occupational therapists, orthotists or prosthetists, rehabilitation doctors and others, as already discussed earlier in this book under "Spinal Injuries". The final aim should be to rehabilitate the patient, not only to the activities of daily living, but also wherever possible to return to some employment. This may mean retraining and adjustments to the place of work and to the home, such as ramps, supporting rails, low benches, together with adjustments and attachments to machines.

All large firms should also be required by law to have a minimum of perhaps 3% of its workforce recruited from those with a significant disability. The needs of the paraplegic and other severely disabled include ramps in public buildings, and special lavatories for the incapacitated.

REHABILITATION

SEVERE INJURIES

Early ← Physiotherapy and Mobility / Occupational Therapy / Rehabilitation

Early → Retraining for Suitable Jobs

AMPUTEES

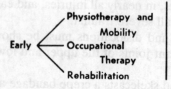

Early Re-education and Mobility

UPPER LIMB

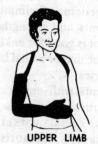

LOWER LIMB

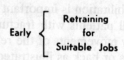

PARAPLEGICS

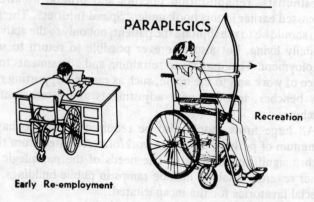

Recreation

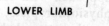

Early Re-employment

REHABILITATION

DAILY LIVING

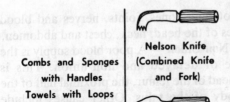

Combs and Sponges
with Handles
Towels with Loops
Bath with Seat
Lavatory Rails

**WASHING
AND TOILET**

Nelson Knife
(Combined Knife
and Fork)

Rubber Handle
on Spoon

EATING

Ground Floor
Ramps and
Suitable Doors
Low Basins
and Stoves

HOUSING

TRANSPORT

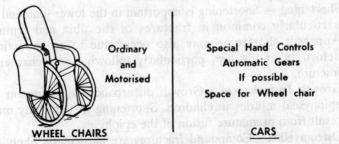

Ordinary
and
Motorised

WHEEL CHAIRS

Special Hand Controls
Automatic Gears
If possible
Space for Wheel chair

CARS

INDUSTRY

Low Benches
Adjusted Controls for Machines
Guards if Necessary

**ADJUSTMENT TO
MACHINES AND BENCHES**

Ramps for Wheel Chairs
Suitable Canteen
and Lavatory Doors

**ADJUSTMENT TO
PREMISES**

GENERAL COMPLICATIONS OF INJURIES

These may involve not only bones, joints, nerves and blood vessels but also injuries of the head, neck, chest and abdomen.

Bones — Delayed and Non-Union — A poor blood supply is the most common cause of delayed and non-union. This is particularly so in the head of the femur, the proximal half of the scaphoid and the body of the talus. Other causes include excessive movement at the fracture site, interposition of soft tissue between bone ends, infections and pathological bone, as in secondary deposits from carcinoma. Over-distraction and operative periosteal stripping may also delay union.

Mal-Union - This is important in the radius and ulna where forearm rotation will be affected. Malalignment of the femur and the tibia may result in osteoarthritis.

Shortening — Shortening is important in the lower limb and is particularly common in fractures of the tibia and femur. Apparent shortening may also occur due to an adduction deformity of the hip, particularly following a trochanteric fracture.

Growth Disturbances - Growth disturbances are common in epiphyseal injuries in children. Shortening or deformity may result from premature fusion of the epiphyses.

Osteomyelitis - Compound fractures are particularly likely to lead to osteomyelitis. This is difficult to treat and may lead to non-union or shortening.

Joints - Stiffness and pain may result from injury to a joint. It is also common following prolonged immobilisation, as in plaster. Prolonged traction on the knee may also lead to pain and swelling of the joint. Joints likely to become stiff include the shoulder and the metacarpo-phalangeal if they are immobilised for more than three weeks, particularly in old people.

GENERAL COMPLICATIONS OF INJURIES

BONES

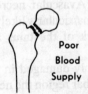

Delayed and Non-Union

Poor Blood Supply

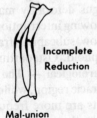

Avascular Necrosis

Incomplete Reduction

Mal-union

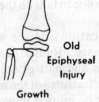

Shortening

Incomplete Reduction

Growth Disturbances

Old Epiphyseal Injury

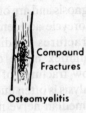

Osteomyelitis

Compound Fractures

JOINTS

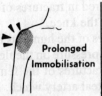

Stiffness and Pain

Prolonged Immobilisation

(P)

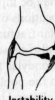

Instability

Old Ligament or Meniscus Injury

(P)

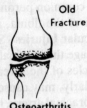

Osteoarthritis

Old Fracture

(P) or (S)

Instability is common in the knee and ankles due to ligamentous injuries and wasting of muscles. Osteoarthritis is common in joints where fractures have been incompletely reduced. Change in weightbearing patterns due to a varus or valgus deformity may also cause arthritis. Avascular necrosis following interruption of the blood supply is particularly likely to follow subcapital fractures of the hip, neck of the talus and scaphoid. Osteoarthritis will follow.

Neurological — **The spinal cord** is commonly damaged in the thoracic region, while in the cervical and lumbar region the nerve roots are more frequently divided.

In the thoracolumbar region, both cord and nerve roots may be damaged.

In the **upper limb**, brachial plexus injuries have a poor prognosis and are often due to falls on the point of the shoulder in motorcycle accidents.

Fractures or dislocations of the shoulder may lead to circumflex nerve damage. Radial nerve injuries commonly follow fractures of the midshaft of the humerus, ulnar nerve paralysis is often due to fractures of the medial epicondyle, while the median nerve may be injured in wrist fractures and lunate dislocations.

In the **lower limb**, the sciatic nerve is commonly damaged in posterior dislocations of the hip and in fractures of the pelvis. The common peroneal nerve may be injured in fractures of the neck of the fibula, and in dislocations of the knee.

Vascular Injuries - Supracondylar fractures of the humerus may damage the brachial artery and also cause pressure on the flexor muscles of the forearm. Supracondylar fractures of the femur, similarly, may cause damage to the popliteal artery which, like the brachial artery, has a poor collateral blood supply. Both may lead to gangrene or muscle ischaemia.

Other Complications - These include those due to tight plasters and traumatic ossification, respiratory obstruction in head, jaw and chest injuries, abdominal and pelvic injuries as well as shock, fat embolus, and the crush syndrome.

GENERAL COMPLICATIONS
OF INJURIES

NERVE INJURIES

	Brachial Plexus Circumflex Radial Ulnar Median	Sciatic Lateral Popliteal
Spinal Cord Damage	Nerves Upper Limb	Nerves Lower Limb

VASCULAR INJURIES

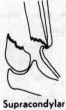 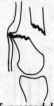

Supracondylar Humerus	Supracondylar Femur	Tight Plaster

OTHER COMPLICATIONS

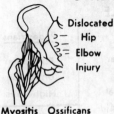

Dislocated Hip Elbow Injury	Head Jaw and Chest Injuries	Gut Spleen Bladder Other Organs
Myositis Ossificans	Respiratory Obstruction	Abdominal and Pelvic Injuries

THE FUTURE
SAFE CARS

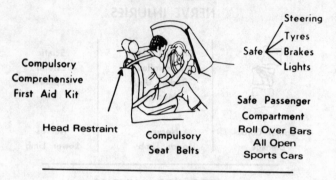

Compulsory
Comprehensive
First Aid Kit

Safe ← Steering / Tyres / Brakes / Lights

Head Restraint

Compulsory
Seat Belts

Safe Passenger
Compartment
Roll Over Bars
All Open
Sports Cars

SAFE ROADS

Centre and Side
Crash Barriers
All Highways

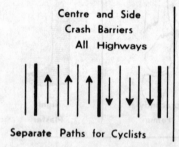

Separate Paths for Cyclists

Surface Road Non Skid
All Roads
Reflectors or
Lighted
Subways for all
Pedestrians
Helicopter Highway
Patrols

SAFE PEOPLE

Drivers

Complete Ban
Alcohol and
Certain Drugs

Car + Drivers

Yearly Test Car
and
Yearly Test ← Medical / First Aid
Driving
Speed Limits

Pedestrians

Forbidden
on Major
Highways

Underpasses
and Footbridges

THE FUTURE
EDUCATION PUBLIC

<u>SAFE TRAVEL</u>	<u>SAFE HOMES</u>	<u>SAFE WORK</u>
Electricity	Factories
Kitchens	and
Non-Skid Floors	Offices
and
Bathrooms

HOSPITALS

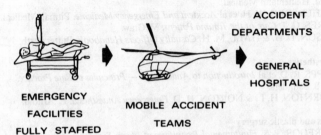

ACCIDENT
DEPARTMENTS

GENERAL
HOSPITALS

EMERGENCY
FACILITIES
FULLY STAFFED

MOBILE ACCIDENT
TEAMS

REGIONALISATION OF ACCIDENT SERVICES

COMPREHENSIVE
ACCIDENT
TRAINING
SURGEONS
DOCTORS
NURSES
AMBULANCE
OFFICERS

DOCTORS

COMPULSORY
ACCIDENT
KITS — CARS
HOMES
OFFICES

ADEQUATE
CONSULTANT
ACCIDENT
SURGEONS

Recommended publications for detailed management of injuries

This list is given only as a guide. There are many excellent publications on all subjects.

Accident surgery
EASTON, K. *Rescue Emergency Care.* Heinemann Medical.
FRAENKEL, G. J. & LUDBROOK, J. *Guide to the House Surgeon in the Surgical Unit.* Heinemann Medical.
RUTHERFORD, W. H. et al *Accident and Emergency Medicine.* Pitman Medical.
SHIRES, G. T. *Care of the Trauma Patient.* McGraw.
WILSON, D. H. & HALL, M. H. *Casualty Officers Handbook.* Butterworth.

Anaesthetics
DRIPPS, R. D. et al *Introduction to Anaesthesia — Principles of Safe Practice.* W. B. Saunders.
THORNTON, H. L. & NORTON, H. D. *Emergency Anaesthesia.* E. Arnold.

Burns and plastic surgery
McGREGOR, I. A. *Fundamental Techniques of Plastic Surgery and their Surgical Applications.* Churchill Livingstone.

Chest injuries
KEEN, G. *Chest Injuries — A Guide for Accident Departments.* Wright.

Fractures and dislocations
ADAMS, J. C. *Outline of Fractures.* Churchill Livingstone.
APLEY, A. G. *A System of Orthopaedics and Fractures.* Butterworths.
CHARNLEY, J. *The Closed Treatment of Common Fractures.* Churchill Livingstone.
ROCKWOOD, C. A. et al *Fractures in Adults and Children.* Lippincott.

Hand injuries
CONOLLY, W. B. & KILGORE, E. S. *Hand Injuries and Infections.* E. Arnold.
FLATT, A. E. *The Care of Minor Hand Injuries.* Mosby.
PARRY, C. B. W. *Rehabilitation of the Hand.* Butterworth.

Head injuries
HAYWARD, R. *Management of Acute Head Injuries.* Blackwell.
POTTER, J. M. *The Practical Management of Head Injuries.* Lloyd-Luke.

Operative surgery
CAMPBELL'S OPERATIVE ORTHOPAEDICS.
Eds. A. S. Edmonson & A. H. Crenshaw, Mosby.
FARQUHARSON, E. L. *Textbook of Operative Surgery.*
Ed. R. R. Rintoul, Churchill Livingstone.
ROB, C. & SMITH, R. *Operative Surgery.* Butterworth.

Spinal injuries
BEDBROOK, SIR GEORGE. *Care and Management of Spinal Cord Injuries.*
Springer Verlag.

Other publications
HUCKSTEP, R. L. *Skelecasts — A Lightweight Concept of Immobilisation.* East
African Medical Journal, **46**, 604.
HUCKSTEP, R. L. *Intramedullary Compression Nail for Femoral Shaft Fractures.*
Journal of Bone and Joint Surgery, **54B**, 204, 384, **61B**, 237, **67B**, 494.
HUCKSTEP, R. L. *Huckstep Intramedullary Nail.* In: *Concepts in Intramedullary
Nailing.* Ed. D. Seligson, Grune & Stratton, 1985.
HUCKSTEP, R. L. *Huckstep Intramedullary Nail.* In: *Clinical Orthopaedics and
Related Research.* Ed. D. Wiss, Lippincott, 1986.
HUCKSTEP, R. L. *Huckstep Intramedullary Compression Nail and Ceramic Hip.*
Downs Surgical, London and Sydney, 1986.
HUCKSTEP, R. L. *Titanium Alloy Circlip for Difficult Oblique Fractures.* Journal
of Bone and Joint Surgery, **62B**, 263.
HUCKSTEP, R. L. *Cementless Ceramic Modular Hip and Femoral Replacement.*
Journal of Bone and Joint Surgery, **66B**, 787.
HUCKSTEP, R. L. *Staple and Screw for Recurrent Dislocation of Shoulder.* Journal
of Bone and Joint Surgery, **65B**, 674, and Downs Surgical, London and Sydney,
1986.
HUCKSTEP, R. L. *Early Mobilisation of Patients with Fractures and Orthopaedic
Conditions.* Australian and New Zealand Journal of Surgery, **47**, 344.
HUCKSTEP, R. L. *Simple Guidelines to Disasters.* Australian Family Physician, **7**,
36.
HUCKSTEP, R. L. *Disaster Plan.* The Prince of Wales/Prince Henry Hospitals,
Sydney.

Emergency management of vehicle accidents

Extinguish cigarettes — Turn off ignition —
Warn oncoming traffic —
Clear airway — Ensure continued air entry and oxygenation —
Stop bleeding — Elevate and splint injured limbs, neck and spine
— Free patient — Look for other casualties — Call for assistance.

Recommended equipment

The following equipment is recommended. The minimum that every person with first aid training should carry is listed below. It is also advised that where possible the additional equipment listed be carried especially in more remote areas.

First aid kit for general use

(In reflective yellow shoulder pack)

1 torch plus 2 batteries
1 lightstick
1 disposable waterproof cape (pocket size)
1 space blanket
6 tie on labels (3 red and 3 green disaster or luggage labels)
1 waterproof felt marking pen
1 pair scissors — all purpose heavy duty
1 whistle
1 small tube handcleaner
6 bandages — triangular
1 roll plaster wool 15 cm
2 cling bandages 15 cm } or 2 large shell dressings
2 cling bandages 10 cm
3 combines (9 × 29 cm)
3 combines (15 × 20 cm)
1 small tin assorted adhesive dressings

1 roll 2.5 cm elastic adhesive bandage
2 airways (disposable) Nos. 2 and 3
1 collapsible face mask (optional)
1 cervical collar — Plastazote or inflatable
1 tube (small) antiseptic anaesthetic cream
First aid manual

Extra for doctors, nurses and paramedics

Stethoscope — lightweight paediatric
4 syringes (2 ml + needles + alcohol wipes + drugs as indicated
    — see below)
2 Dwellcath needles (12G) — for upper tracheal puncture
1 long leg pneumatic splint + 2 malleable splints for arms
1 Entonox (nitrous oxide/oxygen) inhaler
1 spinal board (lightweight)
1 small plastic bowl + paper tissues
1 Velcro tourniquet
Syringe and suction catheter or mini-suction pump and catheter
1 auto inflatable bag and mask for artificial ventilation + 1 adult
    and 1 children's face mask
2 needles through finger stall or with Heimlich valves (for tension
    pneumothorax)
2 plastic cannulae with inserting needles for chest aspiration
Sterile gloves — 2 pairs
Cuffed endotracheal tubes + connections + laryngoscope +
    lubricant
1 oro-nasal tube + syringe
1 urethral catheter
Small hacksaw (15 cm) for emergency amputations (including 2
    sterile blades, 4 artery forceps, 1 scalpel + 2 blades, 1 pair
    scissors, plus suture material dressings + alcohol wipes)

Drugs

2 × 500 ml plasma expander complete with giving set
Aminophylline 250 mg × 5
Lignocaine 2% — 20 ml
Diazepam 10 mg × 2

Sodium bicarbonate 8.4% — 100 ml
Amethocaine eye drops
Pethidine 50 mg × 6
Atropine 500 micrograms × 4
Ketamine 100 mg × 10
Adrenaline 1 in 1000 1 ml × 2
Lignocaine jelly
Sodium versenate (5 ml — dilute in 100 ml) for alkali in eyes
2 plain blood bottles (for blood samples)
Other emergency drugs, e.g. naloxone 0.4 mg × 5 and syrup of
  ipecacuanha B.P. — 100 ml

General car equipment
Four-way indicator flasher switch
1 flashing torch (red with white non-flashing beam)
Reflective number plates
2 reflective danger triangles
Fire extinguisher
Seat belts and head restraint
Map
Car tools, i.e. jack, screwdriver, pliers, adjustable spanner, tyre
  levers, hammer and plastic insulating tape
Hacksaw — small portable + 2 spare blades
Container of water — 2 litres minimum
Small towel or disposable towels or wipes
Penknife — multi-purpose with scissors

Emergency telephone numbers and notes

Emergency telephone numbers and notes

Index